DATE DUE

NO 3 '03		
DE 17 '05		

Woman's Strength

A Woman's Book of Strength

Karen Andes

A PERIGEE BOOK

A Perigee Book
Published by The Berkley Publishing Group
A division of Penguin Putnam Inc.
375 Hudson Street
New York, NY 10014

Copyright © 1995 by Karen Andes
Book design by Irving Perkins Associates
Cover design by James R. Harris.
Cover and interior photographs by Irene Young.
Models: Karen Andes and Nancy Mimms.

First edition: January 1995

The Penguin Putnam Inc. World Wide Web site address is
http://www.penguinputnam.com

Published simultaneously in Canada.

Library of Congress Cataloging-in-Publication Data

Andes, Karen.
A woman's book of strength / Karen Andes.—1st ed.
p.   cm
"A Perigee Book."
Includes bibliographical references.
ISBN 0-399-51899-1 (pbk. : alk. paper)
1. Bodybuilding for women—Psychological aspects.   2. Weight
training for women—Psychological aspects.   I. Title.
GV546.6.W64A53   1995
646.7′5′082—dc20   94-29498
                                                   CIP

Printed in the United States of America

20   19   18   17   16   15   14

This book is printed on acid-free paper.

*This book is dedicated to all women
who, for many reasons, were denied the opportunity to be strong
or never knew the possibility existed.*

*It is meant to inform and remind
those contemplating the path,
and those already on it,
to keep going, even through darkness.*

*And it is my wish
that, in the future, this book may serve
younger generations of women
who won't be afraid
to be strong.*

Gracias

WRITING THIS BOOK has taught me the ultimate lesson that strength doesn't grow without resistance or the support of others. In acknowledging all who believed in me, encouraged me, or put up with me during this process, I begin with those who didn't. The people who told me I "couldn't do it" actually lit an important fire inside me. They helped give me the determination, discipline and sheer stubbornness to see my way through.

But with more affection, I thank those who lifted me up from the beginning: my mother, who gave me a taste for pleasure and the inspiration to live a long, healthy life; my grandmother, who taught me to take pains with each creation, for each is an extension of oneself; my uncle Johnny, who inspired my urge to fly; my sister, Andes Bell, who taught me how to read when I was three and showed me that dancing around the room is one of the best ways to have a good time; and my father, Charles Andes, who has more than once worried about my direction in life but now can rest assured.

I am grateful to my teachers at Solebury School in New Hope, Pennsylvania, especially David Leshan, Julia Moreau and Peter Brodie, who realized that talent in a young girl can be a tougher seed to sprout than in a young boy.

I thank Bill Gifford, my writing teacher from Vassar College, who plucked my short story from a pile of many, and put me into a writing class that changed the direction of my life.

My special thanks to John Irving, who encouraged me long before I knew what it would take to complete a book and who also was the first person to put a dumbbell in my hand.

I am grateful to John Gardner, with whom I studied briefly at Bread Loaf Writers' Conference, two weeks before his death in 1982. His work continues to remind me to keep my writing "moral."

I thank trainers Kirk Miller of New York and Shari Shryock of San Francisco, for teaching me the ropes of bodybuilding, and the International Dance Exercise Association for sponsoring my workshops since 1988, even though what I had to say didn't always fit into the world of aerobic exercise. I thank my friend Ralph Francis, who has been generous with both legal and training advice, and Steve Sisgold for showing me that selling doesn't have to be about oneself but about the message. I'm also grateful to Gold's Gym in Marin, California, where my passion and my investment are tied into one organism, each sustaining the other.

I am grateful to Cher, the tattooed goddess, wild woman of the entertainment business, for choosing me as one of her trainers and letting me live part-time in her house, where I churned out some of the first pages of this book.

I thank my agent, Leslie Keenan, of the Printed Voice, Woodside, California, for believing in this book and finding it a good home at Putnam. I am especially grateful to my editor, Julie Merberg, for "getting" the message of this book and for bringing it out into the world.

Mostly, I thank my husband, Martine Carcamo, who, more than anyone else, has run this whole race with me and been my greatest support. He has taught me how to fix things that are broken and build other things from scratch. At his side, I have ferried over the threshold of youthful impatience into the deep, quiet waters of intimate friendship and a life with more substance.

Finally, I must thank my invisible collaborator. When I tried to write novels, I thought too hard and worked too much yet didn't have much to show for it. I figured there had to be a better way. So I started accessing a different part of my brain and a new voice emerged in my journal writings. This other voice and I don't always agree. She's the one who scoffs at my outlines, spins a simple phrase into a whole new chapter and spills her enthusiasm and poetry where I think it doesn't belong. I'm the one with the agenda, the tension, the deadline, the critical mind. Her job is to run free and sing in whatever crazy voice she wants. My job is to play receiver at the keyboard and not squelch her playfulness while she's in the act. Later, after the work has stewed in the pot for a few weeks or months, I can come in as the ruthless, red-penned critic, and by then we both agree. She then lets me take the credit and cash the checks. Without her high-powered whimsy, this book would have never come to light.

Contents

A Woman Wakes Up   xvii

Part One
The Core

Introduction: Finding Our Way   3
My Life in Motion   9
What Is Strength?   19
Fear of Strength   21
   The Sensuality of Strength   29
Why We Need Strength   31
The Journey In   36
   Slowing Down   38
The Principle of the Iron   41
In Balance: Hard and Soft   43
   In Balance with the Elements   45
      Earth   46
      Water   47
      Fire   48
      Air   49

Part Two
The Mechanics

Transformation Begins in Posture   53
   The Weight Training Posture   54
   The Body's Core   55

Core Stabilizing Exercises 55

Neutral Spine 57

Posture Details 57

Align the Body in a Cross 60

The Vertical Line 60

The Horizontals 61

The "Whole" Body 61

Intelligent Use of the Forces   63

Gravity 63

Three Types of Lifts 63

Every Joint Is a Pulley 66

The Underlying Geometry 68

Lines 68

Arcs 72

Which Comes First: Compounds or Isolations? 73

Levers 74

What Is Full Range of Motion? 75

Avoid the Dead Zone 75

Momentum 75

Give Muscles a Full Menu 76

Reps, Sets, Weight and All That Jazz   77

Good Pain, Bad Pain 77

The Quality of Repetitions 78

How Many Reps? 79

Counting 79

How Many Sets? 80

How Many Exercises? 81

Order of Exercises 81

Fast Twitch/Slow Twitch—Muscle Fibers in Action 82

Rep Speeds 83

  2 Up, 4 Down 83

  The 10-Second Rep 83

  10 Down, Explode on 1 84

Half-Reps & Holds 84

A Good Fail 85

Breathing 86

Stretch Between Sets 86

Periodization 87

The Splits   87
    The Basic Beginner, Whole Body Workout   88
    A Standard Advanced Beginner Split   88
    The Basic Three-Day Split   88
    A Four-Day Split   89
    A Quirky Five-Day Split (My Split)   89
    Opposing Muscle Groups   90
    An "On the Run" Split (Catch It When You Can)   90
Aerobics and Training   91
Go Out and Play   92
Plateaus and Valleys   93
What You Can Expect on This Journey: Romance and Commitment   94

Self-Assessment: The Body Puzzle   **99**
Evaluations   99
Posture   101
Some Postural Fixes   103
Muscle Checklist   105

Part Three
The Exercises

The Shifting Truth   **111**
How to Choose Exercises from This Book   112
Exercise Symbol Key   113

Leg Exercises   **116**
Leg Press   116
Sit-Back Squats   118
Lunges   120
Leg Extension with Machine and Ankle Weights   122
Hack Squat   124
Reverse Hack Squat   126
"Stiff" Legged Deadlifts   128
Inner Thigh with Machine, Cables and Ankle Weights   130
Hip Extension with Cables and Ankle Weights   132
Multi-Hip Machine   134
Standing Hamstring Curls with Machine and Ankle Weights   136
Prone Hamstring Curl   138

Leg Raises with No Weight or Ankle Weight 140

Calf Exercises   **142**

Toe Press on Leg Press Machine 142

Seated Calf Raise 144

Standing Calf Raise 146

Back Exercises   **148**

Pull-Downs to Chest 148

Straight Arm Pull-Downs 150

One-Arm Row with Dumbbell or Cable 152

Seated Cable Row 154

Lower Back Hyperextension 156

Chest Exercises   **158**

Bench Press 158

Dumbbell Flye 160

Standing Cable Crossovers (or Cable Flyes) 162

Shoulder Exercises   **164**

Lateral Raises 164

Shoulder Presses 166

Front Cable Raise 168

Half Upright Rows 170

Rear Delt Variations 172

External & Internal Rotators 174

Biceps Exercises   **176**

Barbell Curl 176

Dumbbell Curl 178

Incline Cable Curl 180

Preacher Curls 182

Triceps Exercises   **184**

Press-Downs 184

Dumbbell Triceps Extension 186

French Press 188

Triceps Kickback 190

Abdominal Exercises   **192**

Reverse Curls 192

Rollbacks 194

Good Old Crunches 196

Stretches   **198**

Sample Workouts   **202**

Beginner Workouts 203
    Full Body Workout #1 203
    Full Body Workout #2 204
    Sample Beginner Weekly Menu 204
Intermediate Workouts 205
    Back and Biceps 205
    Legs 205
    Chest, Shoulders, Triceps 206
    Sample Intermediate Weekly Menu 206
Advanced Workouts 207
    Back, Rear Delt, Abs 207
    Quads, Inner Thigh, Calves 207
    Chest and Shoulders 208
    Buttocks, Hamstrings, Outer Thigh 208
    Arms and Abs 209
    Sample Advanced Weekly Menu 209

Part Four

The Rewards of Practice: Heart, Mind & Future

Transcendental Repetitions   **213**
    "Framing" 213
    Ground and Center 216
    Journey into the Soul of a Transcendental Set 217
    The Pleasure of Partnering 220
    A Good Spot 221
    Gym Etiquette 222
Working Out with "Difficult" Emotions   **223**
    Sadness/Depression 224
    Vulnerable/Hurting 225
    Fear 226
    Anger 227
    Tired 227
    Rest 228
The Power Zone   **229**
    Ordinary Magic 232

Approaching Mastery   **233**
And on into the Future 235

Part Five
Food, Tools and Toys

Easy, Low-Fat, Old-World Recipes for Hectic, Modern Times **241**
Fat 243
Protein 244
Carbohydrates 244
Stocking the Kitchen 245
Substitution 247
A Day in the Life 247
Recipes 251
 Gallo Pinto or Fancy Rice and Beans 251
 Turkey Burgers 253
 Karen's Incredible Caesar Salad 254
 Egg White Fritata 256
 Pasta Con Frijoles 257
Foods to Eat When You're on the Go 259
Maintenance Tips 259
It's a Jungle Out There 260
Meditation for the Fully Realized Woman **263**
More Tools and Toys for Transformation **264**
Also by Karen 265
 Deep-Water Aquatic Exercise 265
 More Aquatic Equipment 265
Videos 266
Inversion Equipment 266
References **267**
The Body 267
The Mind 268
The Evolution of Spirit 268
Women 268
Food 268

A Woman Wakes Up

A woman wakes up to the world,
    Awed by the vastness
    Outside her and within.
    She starts seeing patterns take shape in her life,
    Hears rhythms emerge from the mystery,
    Feels forces at work around her,
    But doubts their presence and herself.
    Messages sail forward in the night,
    Artfully wrapped in dreams.
    But throughout the day, she loses touch,
    Forgets what she knows, who she is,
    And what she came to do.

She longs to be let in on the secrets
    Of how things work
    And to find her missing pieces.
    She is driven but doesn't know why
    To weave, sculpt, sing, and lay down histories,
    To make gardens, children, fortunes,
    Herself into a work of art.
    But where does she begin?

She has bounced between indulgence and strict vows of cleansing,
    Flying high and hungry,
    Proud of her brief victory over emptiness.

But her dry mouth and brittle-bone weakness,
Cry for sweetness, satisfaction, a compassionate touch,
And all resolutions crumble.
She sees only imperfection, not the rebel soul demanding time.

She studies, reads, takes seminars in self-improvement,
Delivers herself to be analyzed,
Charting her course by stars, instincts, the counsel of others.
Broken pieces begin to mend.
Untamed parts of her personality venture back into the corral.
Old pains that used to leave her flattened, slowly disappear.
Yet other parts still drift on an open sea . . .
Anchored to nothing, heading nowhere,
Sometimes anxious to be claimed,
Other times, wanting no structure or direction.

She shares dessert with a friend
Whose insights carry the chill of truth:
"Clear away the noise, shame and fear,
Even the *aspirations*,
That have pushed you into frenzies," she says.
"Pulled you off in ten directions,
Away from your core.
Your beauty is pulsing under the surface,
Waiting for a safe time to come out.
Simply create a sacred place for it, silence.
Get up before dawn or burn the candle late if you must.
Tap the knowing that comes from the belly—not the brain.
Understand, there is a greater source, gentler than the will, ego or
the need to survive.
Believe, and when you're ready, surrender . . ."

What does it all mean, she wonders?
What catapulting action? What violent unknown?
What should she do—pull up roots or put them down?
Quit her job and sail off in a new direction? Or follow the course
she's on?
Finally, with nothing but courage to guide her,
She makes a move, a phone call, a declaration,

A promise to honor this voice that says, "Be as you are in your
    wishes.
Waste no more time."
And so, she jumps,
Feet upended,
Petticoat flying,
With no obvious destination in sight,
Tumbling into her wishes, her body, her every illogical desire,
Falling,
Floating,
Then flying—
Even banking through the turns
Just as she does in her dreams.

The rhythms she has heard and doubted
    Start pounding in her ear.
Patterns take on color, shadow and dimension.
Words flow in a voice she didn't know she had.
She comes alive in the warm, welcoming interiors of her flesh and
    muscle,
Moving on the joy that floods from her heart.
Where she thought she was fixed, she is supple,
Shifting like clay under a new loving touch.

But every day there is that risk of separation,
    Of losing what she's after,
Faltering under the demands of time or her own compulsive desires.
Every day she needs reminders:
A journal full of dreams,
A grounding stone in her pocket,
A silken box of found treasures, others passed by on the street.
A word,
A deep breath,
A belly laugh,
Bare feet in the earth
And friends on a similar journey.

Day after day, she returns to herself for magic
    Or the world becomes flat and dry.

Her inner life is lush, private—a hidden garden
She strolls through daily, noting the weeds and wild, blooming
    orchids,
The crops she put in last season,
The seedlings that sprouted overnight.
She learns to see without praise or condemnation
And soon finds herself reflected in everything around her—
Even the charred half of a pine tree, sliced by lightning,
Rotting on the forest floor, now a home to ants and beetles
With its good side standing strong, spitting out pine cones and
    oozing sap.

A strange transformation has taken place.
What brings pleasure is not a bauble or the promise of reward but
    the work itself.
Her treasures are the tiniest details:
A warm teacup cradled in both hands,
The rising sun,
The scent of jasmine,
The steady engine of strength that purrs inside her,
Roosters breaking the silence,
Though she has been awake for hours.

Part One

The Core

Introduction:
Finding Our Way

"There was one spot that was unique, a spot where I could be at my very best. It was my job to distinguish it from all other places."

CARLOS CASTANEDA: *The Teachings of Don Juan*

EVERY DAY IN THE GYM, I see more of them. They seem to wash in with the tide—shy newcomers in baggy T-shirts, clutching a workout card as if it were a map to a foreign country. They wander among the machinery trying to look inconspicuous and figure out what to do. By the looks on their faces, I can see they don't know a dumbbell from a barbell or a set from a rep. I want to give suggestions and encouragement. But I've learned from experience not to offer my services unsolicited. So instead I watch and sometimes cringe at the way they tackle the exercises without much sensitivity, inward connection or obvious enjoyment. And I know chances are good that when the next tide washes out, they'll float out with it and I'll never see them again.

I've often wondered what it would take to change this. Ideally, I'd like to sit each woman down and find out what brought her here. I want to know what she wants for herself, what she does for a living, how much time she doesn't have, if she's got kids, a mate, a history of athleticism, any old injuries to be aware of, what she ate for dinner last night, lunch, breakfast, how she feels when she looks in the mirror and how many voices run the show inside her head. If she'd let me, I'd study her posture to see where she's rigid, collapsed or off-center—a clue to where she carries her pain—and swap some of my own tales of being twisted, numb, shapeless and weak before I began strengthening my body with weights at age 30. I'd like to show her how to make changes without feeling burdened by an impossible ideal—or pushed into exercise by guilt and fear. Ultimately, I'd like to present this experience as pleasure, a sanctuary from outside cares and her chance to take up the chisel and reshape both her body and mind.

Yet, nine times out of ten, I know she's going to say, "But I don't want big muscles. I just want to get rid of this." (I note the phrase "get rid of" as if it were garbage.) I could give her the standard "don't worry" speech:

"Most women can't grow big muscles," I'd explain, "because they don't have enough male hormones. Most of the big women you see in muscle magazines took steroids to get that way. But natural women's muscles grow very slowly. In fact, even after years of training, our muscles don't increase much in size—although they get stronger, shapelier and, when body fat is low, more defined."

But by this time, I may have lost her. The words have to be ones she can actually *hear* and therefore, can help her launch her dreams. But "size" and even "definition" are dry, foreign and don't stir most women's passions. I'm certainly careful to avoid "bulk up" or even "bodybuilding" since these tend to be a real turn-off and not what she's after. If I play it safe and use neutral phrases from exercise physiology, such as "muscle diameter," "lean tissue" and "fat-to-muscle ratio," I place a technical boundary between us. Yet, just as I consider her, I also avoid phrases that bother *me*—patronizing, polite "ladies' " terms, as in "This one firms the tummy, ladies" or self-abusive gym lingo such as "This blasts the butt," both of which perpetuate stereotypes I'm trying to break. I may try words such as "sleek," "elegant," "graceful" and "sexy," but even these don't describe the whole picture because they don't include the internal process I'm also trying to present. It would be simpler if I could just grab her by the hand and say, "Come with me. This is good."

This journey into strength is not just about sculpting the body but how we can use the *pathway* of our bodies as a way to mine the strength in ourselves. For when external and internal strength are blended and balanced, the wires connect, the whole person wakes up and that union of flesh and spirit is magnificent, radiant, a cause to rejoice!

For so many women, this pursuit of strength is new, awkward, controversial, even frightening. Many of us are still afraid of who we might alienate if we get *too* strong, and simultaneously afraid of the dark, dangerous fates that await us if we don't get strong *enough*. Or we may think that, in order to be strong, we have to sacrifice our fragile natures, become more like men, change the fundamental structure of who we are. Yet we can't just put on the cloak of male strength and strut around. It doesn't feel right because we didn't create it—we might as well wear their shoes. We need to approach this on our own terms, using our own vocabulary if we need to, taking our own time—even if the methods we use are basic and also used by men.

It would help if we had more role models. But there aren't many—maybe an ancient goddess or two, a professional athlete, a movie star, Wonder Woman—few *real* women with lives like ours, who juggle responsibilities yet make time for a physical discipline, and spark in others the thought, "Well, if she can do it, so can I."

Starting this journey takes courage. It's not easy to be a beginner and embark on something that could take a while. It requires keen vision to see beyond all the conflicting information out there, the jumble of various body ideals, and pierce through to the truth of what we want and how to get it. And it takes time invested to understand that the real trophies of strength aren't found in strong muscles or winning competitions, but in the discipline of practice.

Why do we want strength anyway? It's not for physical perfection—thank God many of us have let *that* one go. No, we are women of action, ability and substance and simply want a physical body that reflects how we feel inside. We have healthy appetites, sensual flesh. We don't relate to the timid, anorexic-looking waifs that flood the fashion pages—and we certainly don't want to be the She-Hulk either. We want a body that will see us through decades of activity and still looks good at sixty, seventy, eighty and beyond. And if it jiggles in certain places, so be it. We celebrate ourselves, regardless. However, the longer we keep up this discipline, the greater the chance we'll get what might have gotten us started in the first place—tight buttocks, chiseled abdominals, strong upper bodies, muscle that ripples when we move.

Strong muscles aren't just cosmetic. The truth is, we *need* strength, perhaps even more than men do since it helps us fight some of our more difficult, feminine-based struggles with ourselves. When our muscles are stronger, our metabolisms speed up, which helps keep body fat down. Without even moderate muscle strength, our skeletons sag, our posture crumples and therefore our stature tumbles as well. Over time, as muscles get weak, our bones weaken, too. After menopause, when our calcium-producing ability drops off sharply, we find ourselves at risk for osteoporosis—which becomes more severe if we haven't kept our bones strong all along. Why settle for this when we can do something about it? Weakness takes a psychological toll as well—compounding feelings of helplessness, fear, flagging self-esteem.

There are three key elements to getting and staying strong and lean: muscular strength, aerobic exercise and steady eating habits with low-fat foods. Of the three, creating strength is the most complex, requiring the most detailed attention to posture, form, amount of weight and reps, and so forth. It's also the most misunderstood—which is why I wrote this book. But it won't work alone—and neither will any one or two of the three elements. It has to be all three. Therefore, it may call for a *gradual* shift in habits or creative scheduling. Obsession is not necessary. The time required isn't impossible—just an hour a day of exercise, sometimes less, sometimes more.

The type of strength I present here certainly isn't the stereotypical, ball-breaking, emasculating force conjured up by Amazon-fearing warriors—or by centuries of men after that. It doesn't intend to threaten or intimidate. In fact, its purpose is just the opposite. It's a compassionate, life-sustaining concept, a blend of warmth, kindness and security, for we are mothers, nurturers, lovers, creators, supple creatures who bend with the wind, defenders of the weak, feelers of deep emotion, seekers of truth, even the uncomfortable truth in ourselves. We also have boundaries, ethics, justified rages and we know when to say no. Strong, we inspire change, justice, enlightenment. Weak, the flame inside us dies. Our generation is lucky to have a good picture of "health" and "self-reliance" and to know how to put it into practice. We can truly take the evolution of women forward a notch and pass on the benefits to other women, children and men.

Too many of us have been victims. We can recite in exquisite detail all the dramas and traumas that flattened us in the past—and we know every horrible little thing that's "wrong" with our bodies. But we aren't so eloquent about our ordinary and extraordinary powers, the beauty and magic we already possess. Deep inside, we may sense its presence but we don't know how to bring it out and use it. We're shy about it—and schooled not to be boastful. But this "magic power" is a secret we possess, a bit of whimsy, a flair, our uniqueness, and the very thing that makes us know we're special. It's also the root of our strength, the key to our creativity and our best tool for making ourselves strong. This quality is like a muscle. With practice and attention, it too, can be strong.

This, therefore, is a woman's book of strength as it makes sense to us and addresses both the contours of our bodies and our inner worlds. The type of strength addressed here cuts to all levels—heart, mind, spirit and body—and can be exercised in any area of life where resistance is met. But the work begins in the physical and remains firmly rooted there because in the world of matter and flesh, there is proof. The laws of cause and effect are *visible*—reflecting who and how we are on any given day. We need physical proof because our faith is often weak. Intangibles don't always reassure us. We need something tangible. The results that show up in our bodies reveal the power of our thoughts and actions.

I have written this book for women because most weight training books simply advise readers how to put on muscle *mass*. Here, it's safe to say that size is not the Holy Grail we seek. From an exercise point of view, however, this isn't just a women's book. Honestly, I don't see a difference between women's and men's exercises because we're all dealing with the same laws of physics and most everyone is working with two arms, two legs and a torso. Although women have slightly different body compositions from men, the mechanics of motion are much the same. So, actually, the training information (and much of the internal information) can be just as valuable to men. But I wrote this for women so I could have the freedom to look beyond the issue of muscle mass and address our vulnerability, our rich emotional lives, our sense of self, who we yearn to be (and why) and our quest for self-knowledge.

We're lucky that many of us are novices with weights. This makes us better students, blank slates, free from the burden of pride or past performance. We don't bring with us crusty old training methods and long-ingrained bad form or egos that need reassurance from hurling around heavy iron.

We don't need to have had an athletic background, and it doesn't even matter if we hated school gym class or all types of sports. There's no ball to put in a hoop, no opponent to fight (except oneself.) No one wins, loses or even keeps score. We don't even need to be strong since effective weight lifting requires less strength than sensitivity. And since muscles respond the same way throughout our lives, we can start this sport and benefit from it at any age.

To understand and master the practice of weight training, we must learn slowly. If, in fact, we *could* get the results we wanted tomorrow, we would have learned nothing and would take no satisfaction in our work. In our "gotta have it now" culture, I'd get much richer if I sold fat-melting cream or pills that build muscle while you sleep. But weight training is the only way I know and trust that creates both dramatic short-term and lasting changes—and can also help make us wise.

Finding our way isn't done quickly or easily. It takes some searching and discomfort. And some days, perhaps for weeks at a time, we may see nothing at all. Off days, inconsistency and low energy are part of the formula and have to be figured in. Yet if we can return to our practice—especially on those days—and find our sense of play, then we feed our souls as well. Boredom, in fact, should be seen not as an adversary but a call to creativity, a message from the imagination saying, "Look, you've got to make this interesting for me or I quit." Some of the best discoveries are made on off days.

This journey may feel scary at times when we think we're traveling into the unknown. Yet everything to find here is something we may already know but have forgotten. This guidebook, therefore, points in the same direction for everybody. Its intention is to lead us back to ourselves.

My Life in Motion

MOVEMENT HAS BEEN my longtime companion and best teacher. Throughout my life, it has rescued me from self-destruction, guided me toward health and delivered me to parts of myself I didn't know were there. It continues to give me a precise and immediate reading on my state of mind and reminds me to embrace the subtlety of every step—to be engaged in my life so it doesn't just go by. I'm on my knees with gratitude that I've kept this part of myself alive.

As a child, I liked unstructured movement with no rules: climbing monkey bars, thrusting myself into leaf piles, doing flips and swan dives into the pool, storm-trooping the neighborhood on bikes and dancing all the parts of *Gypsy* and *West Side Story* with my older sister. I liked cartwheels and tumbling. But gym class took the fun out of it all—the trauma of dodgeball leaving red welts on my flesh, the humiliation of the rope climb with weenie arms. Competition made me nervous. Having to be faster than anyone else or keep the ball inside the lines cramped my movement style.

I still prefer motion that inspires expression and doesn't have to please a judge or win a game. I like moving to syncopated rhythms: boogie-woogie, samba, blues piano, a tapping foot, the flow of words, any pattern or tempo my body can catch like a wave. I don't like speeds that take me out of control: mountain biking down steep, rocky slopes or speed-demon downhill skiing. I'm uncomfortable flailing in the back row of a dance class, unable to follow the teacher. I don't use motion to prove something or just get to my destination. I prefer to use motion for the journey itself.

I didn't come from a family of deliberate movers or athletes, although some had the potential. Movement got a job done. It helped weed the garden, wash the car, or it existed as pure recreation—a walk around the block, a game of golf. But it was never revered as an essential part of life (the way I now see it), as crucial as air, water and food.

My mother had the potential. She would have been a powerful swimmer with those square shoulders she had, a decent tennis player with some practice, an elegant body builder with her great legs. But that wasn't part of her world or even part of the thinking back then. I'm not so sure it ever occurred to her. Nice women didn't bother with things like that—oh, maybe a light swim or a halfhearted jog.

But this was the Philadelphia suburbs in the early 60's. We didn't know any women who lifted weights or ran around in a sweat. Even if we had, I'm not sure we'd have given them much respect. The cultivation of a woman's physical energy and strength wasn't highly valued back then. The athletic body type certainly wasn't the ideal of women like my mother, who modeled herself as a kind of hybrid Marilyn Monroe, Grace Kelly and Jackie Kennedy—sensual and physical but without any obvious gristle.

My mother liked to wear dresses that showed off her full figure. She liked to skinny-dip on thick August nights and dance around the living room to Harry Belafonte records. She longed for the promise of tropical beaches, warm breezes, the freedom to cast off whatever it was that shackled her.

Then, when winter clamped down and our skin turned white she would put on ten to twenty pounds and be distant, depressed, corralled by we didn't know what, although now I suspect it was her body and something inside her going unexpressed. I'm not sure a run around the neighborhood, a weight lifting session or a swim at the Y would have completely conquered her weight problems or lifted her sadness. But I suspect they would have helped. They certainly help me.

I remember her litany of weight loss treatments: liquids for breakfast and lunch, grapefruits and a steak for dinner, diet pills from the fat doctor and then the way we'd all "be bad" together, eating hamburgers, French fries, hot fudge sundaes. I suspect this song of denial and indulgence has been sung a thousand times. But back then, we didn't know better.

I'm sure if my mother had lived longer she would have evolved with the rest of us, benefiting from the now basic knowledge about exercise and nutrition. But in her own time, she never got her chance to balance the hungers of her body with those from her soul.

My grandmother, Mimi, on the other hand, never seemed to struggle with her body or the yearnings from her soul. She always seemed to know exactly who she was. She lived next door, and so her influence on us was as strong as the Southern accent that stuck with her, even after sixty years north of the Mason-Dixon line. Her presence next door added history, three generations piggybacked on adjacent lots of land. But her impeccable way of life highlighted our crude approach next door. We ate TV dinners, licked our fingers, ate too fast and laughed too loud. She used sugar tongs on the Saccharin that sat in a little blue glass bowl and always chose the right fork. Her dress size never crept above eight; her feet were an impossible size four, and her bureau drawers were full of pair after pair of full-length, white kid gloves with mother-of-pearl buttons that fastened at the wrist. She identified, I believe, more with her Southern heritage, antiques and clothes than with her body. It was almost as if she didn't even *have* a body or any sensual hungers at all. She seemed to float through her life, like a superior sort of being, fueled only by a cup of Sanka and a scrap of toast, always doing something for somebody, making baby blankets for neighbors, flowers for the church altar, sewing curtains or party dresses to add elegance to every gathering.

I was my mother's daughter—stuck on the sensual plane—but I had yearnings for Mimi's ability to rise above it all. . . .

We suffered a series of fatalities. My parents divorced when I was four. I grew up hearing whispers about aunts and uncles with depression, drinking problems, money problems, cancer. One of my distant uncles went into the cellar one morning and shot himself in the mouth. My grandfather dropped dead at the office.

But when my Uncle Johnny's plane was shot down in Viet Nam in 1966, that was the worst blow of all. He was Mimi's son, my mother's baby brother, my hero and first love, our wild bird, free spirit who, when he did aerial acrobatics or parachuted into the backyard, lived the thrill for each of us. He was our one representative of the magnificent urge to move, to transcend gravity and the boundaries of decorum and human flesh—and fly.

He was in the crew of a rescue plane, serving out his third tour of duty, when the plane was shot down over the Gulf of Tonkin in 1966. No wreckage or bodies were ever found. For eight torturous years, we didn't know if he was dead or a prisoner—in fact, we still don't know. He was only declared "presumed dead." We hope he was killed instantly.

Nothing in our upbringing prepared us to deal with this. I watched Mimi and my mother pour quiet grief into flowerbeds, but there was no outlet for full expression—no designated free zone where it was safe to cry out loud, show the full extent of our despair or, God forbid, any joy. Instead, we held it in, carried on hope, kept his car oiled and his sport jackets wrapped in blue cellophane, hanging in the closet in suspended animation. Every four months we sent packages to "Camp of Detention, US Pilots, Hanoi," with Band-Aids, medicated foot powder, throat lozenges, Chinese Checkers, delousing shampoo, toffee candies, a deck of playing cards, paper and pens, clean underwear, warm socks, Life Savers . . .

Although no one said anything, I got the impression that it wasn't okay anymore to run around the neighborhood. So when I had the urge to move, I kept it hidden, like a stash. I would dance alone in the living room for hours, listening to John Coltrane and the Moody Blues. With movement, it seemed I could dance right out of the confines of my life. I could separate myself from the budding confusion of my sexuality, levitate above the entrapment of my adolescent body, kick it into the corner like a pair of sweaty leotards and split my skin.

In school, however, under the instruction of teachers and coaches, movement was acceptable. I played field hockey and basketball, and in the summer joined the swim team. But my imagination was captured in dance. I studied Martha Graham technique, wore footless tights, and choreographed little pieces I performed. I also studied ballet, though I didn't have the right body for it. My shoulders were too big, my legs too fleshy. I wasn't gaminlike or lighter than air and the turn out of my hips (one measure of success in ballet) was so meek the teacher used to wrap me with a cane. But dance was a world that soothed me, beckoned me, where there was nothing ugly or overtly painful. I always felt safe, and still do, in the confines of a dance studio. The floors and mirrors create a blank space where anything is possible.

When I was sixteen, my mother got cancer of the colon. In the course of three years, she went from tan and riding high in her new home, second marriage and brand-new career selling real estate, to jaundiced yellow, bloated, too weak to move. My stepfather took it upon himself to act as her doctor, and lied to her and us about the seriousness, saying hepatitis was the cause of her yellow color. He let her think that a colostomy was an unnecessary "insurance policy," and so she refused to have one, saying she'd never get to wear a bikini again. Because of the withheld truth, there was never any discussion about death, no fears allowed a voice, no insightful bedside talks about how she had lived her life or what I ought to do with mine, no acceptance, no closure. She didn't even write a will.

After her death, I had a big hole in me that seemed to last for years. My movement life all but disappeared. Nothing could relieve the emptiness, yet I tried, frantically to fill up the space with marijuana, scotch on the rocks, cookies, men. I tried an occasional dance class, too, and brief spurts at running, but couldn't sustain them. Yet even through the blur of unconsciousness, I noticed that without movement, my addictions had a stronger hold on me—and the stronger my addictions, the less desire or ability I had to move.

In my early twenties, I had no sense of anything lasting; I felt rootless. I spent my time quickly building structures and tearing them down, as if to test my resilience, see how well I could survive and on how little. It was as if I had leaks throughout my whole being, no borders around the sacred parts of who I was, and so I let in strangers and dangerous substances, without honoring who I was or what I was creating.

Within two years after graduating from college, I got married, got a prestigious, low-paying job with a magazine, then divorced, quit the job, and decided to follow a dream of writing novels and dancing. So I got a waitress job. All these fast, sweeping actions were motivated by fear—fear of nothingness, loneliness and starvation crashing head-on into my other fears of stagnation, confinement, dreams dying on the vine. But the urge to move was my salvation, the healthy part of myself knocking on the door. Even though I stayed in my cloud of marijuana for a few years, occasionally dancing around the living room to my stoned, private rhythms, it only took me so far and then dumped me there. To go further, to get better, I'd need all my senses. So eventually I gave it up.

During that time, I hacked away at a novel, served a thousand brunches and studied jazz dance in grungy studios above Times Square. I even went to auditions to be a Vegas showgirl and to ride elephants in the circus, but soon learned that making a living at dance depended on whether or not someone else deemed me worthy, and I hated that. And the novel (and the next one) went nowhere . . .

Divorced and displaced by choice, I lived in a $100-a-month room in a boarding house in Brooklyn, sharing a bathroom with a carpenter and a longshoreman. There was a health club half a block away, and so for a free membership and to use the locker room, I started teaching exercise classes at $6 an hour.

This was back before aerobics was a common word, before Jackie, Judi and Jane hit the scene—and certainly before any of us teachers knew what we were doing. Coming from dance, I thought exercise was simple, but in fact it was far more complex. I was impressed with the way women delivered themselves like pilgrims, as if to say, "Take me, mold me, make me better." It was a bigger responsibility than I realized.

There we were, exhilarated with sweat and Donna Summer blaring on the turntable, enacting a ritual that wiped away all our outside distinguishing features, our careers, our families, the lives we'd so carefully constructed or deconstructed. All of that disappeared in the preciousness of the moment. It was a rich, new world. But then after a few years, that type of motion wasn't enough. It didn't shape my body into what I yearned it to be; it didn't speak to my soul.

When I saw bodybuilder Cory Everson win her first Ms. Olympia (on ABC's *Wide World of Sports*), something primal stirred inside me. Here was a type of beauty I'd never seen before. Here was something I could create myself. I didn't have to buy it, be lucky enough to be born into it or have someone deem me worthy. All I had to do was work at it. But where to begin?

None of my dancing or exercise classes prepared me for the head-on confrontation with the inert, always victorious, cool world of dumbbells and barbells. They showed up my weaknesses every time—not just in my body but in my impatience and my willful nature that wanted results, perfection *now*.

I didn't know how to confront my fragility. For years, I'd managed to avoid it. Here was a type of movement that didn't take me *out* of myself but immersed me *in* myself and at first, this was frightening. What I soon discovered was that whole parts of my body had fallen asleep. I couldn't even flex the muscles in my hips, buttocks, inner thigh, chest, shoulders, biceps and triceps—almost everywhere! What I thought I needed was an excavation, to "get in there" with sticks of dynamite, a jackhammer, blow myself up and start again. Really what I needed was compassion, a delicate rewiring of the whole system!

I'd always thought of myself as strong, but the type of strength I had was defensiveness, a mask on my weakness. I was annoyed with my delicate self. After nine months, I still couldn't bench press the humble 45-pound bar and had to call for help to get it off my chest. And the 35-degree scoliosis or "S" curve in my spine made it impossible to put any weight on my shoulders. Therefore, I couldn't squat or lunge with a free bar, do military presses over my head, or even any standing calf raises with weight on my shoulders. In fact, there were more exercises I couldn't do than those I could.

For a while, I tried to "blitz" and "blast" my way through the exercises, as it said in the muscle magazines, where beating yourself into shape seemed to be the norm. I found myself weeding through the contradictions of trainers, gym rats, supplement hawkers, even the various body ideals of women, trying to find the truth that applied to me. But this world I'd just entered was full of illusions, airbrushed photos, drug use, false promises and competition results that lasted just one day. Nonetheless, there had to be *something* here that could help change (as I saw it then) my poochy stomach, flat butt, flabby thighs and puny biceps. If I'd been younger and more impressionable, I might have sold my soul and the functional life of my liver for the short-term hardness, muscle boost and definition I would have gotten from Anovar (an anabolic steroid, popular with women at that time). Several people suggested I try it.

I worked with two good trainers who taught me some fundamentals about form. From there, I was on my own, reading, studying, copying people who looked like they knew what they were doing.

At this same time, I started dabbling in Chinese martial arts. I soon got to a point where I felt I needed to make a decision between weight training and martial arts—because I only had so much time or attention to give each one. The martial arts had its tradition that dated back thousands of years, its promise of wisdom and internal well-being, its wise masters and enormous mysteries. Bodybuilding had none of that. Comparatively speaking, bodybuilding was new and brash, and many of those who were held up as masters were in fact very young and had taken drugs to get that way. There was *some* mystery to it all, but no promise of wisdom or centuries-old tradition that begged my respect. Much of it seemed built on vanity and a need to be different, get attention. I chose bodybuilding because it offered me room for individual expression and could be created anew, though I was a bit embarrassed about what this choice said about me.

I soon discovered that the only way I could "move into" the exercises and command the muscles was to train in very slow motion. To my surprise, that's when my body started waking up. Compared to the macho, "come on, drive it up" style I saw around me, my method seemed too "Zen" to really work, and I often doubted my approach. Yet, when I tested myself with heavy weight, I could lift a lot without cheating. The strength I was building was "true." I wasn't hurting myself and, to my surprise, after three years, my scoliosis straightened out by 20 degrees.

My outer strength was coming along fine, but my inner strength was just taking root. I still had "leaks" in my being and "loose borders" around the sacred parts of myself. In my early thirties I uprooted from the east and moved to California, entered a hasty and immature second marriage, got a nasty divorce and cast to the wind all my writing ambitions—because the passion didn't come from my heart, but from a desire to be admired and make money. I'd been courting illusions, and suddenly everything fell apart. It was a humbling time, capped off by Mimi's death. (She, too, had cancer of the colon but died from a heart attack.) This series of soul-tests seemed to say, "You're not nearly as strong as you think you are."

I looked at my life and saw ruins once again, felt that I was nothing, had nothing, except this daily practice that I performed with weights—which wasn't valued highly by others and which I myself didn't understand. When a pap smear came back questionable, causing the fear that this time the cancer was in me, reality cracked its whip over my head and posed the questions, "What are you doing with your life?" and "What do you really want?" What I wanted were the simple things I could create myself—nice clean movements, steady progress, discipline that would reassure me that I could rely on myself. I wasn't so interested in chasing big dreams. I was much more fascinated by the actual steps it would take to get there. I didn't want to run on fear or illusion or escape the feelings that gushed through me like a waterfall. I wanted to be present. Starting with that, I could go anywhere, do anything I wanted.

The pap smear checked out fine. But I felt as though I'd been given a new life. I began to see that I could apply the same lessons of the weights to creating inner strength as well. Little by little, just as I had built my body, I could wake up distant places in my mind and confront my self-defeating behaviors and unconscious, defensive reactions. I could practice patience, sit with discomfort just a little longer, as if I had a weight on my chest, see the patterns of behavior that were keeping me "small" and afraid of my life, of my overpowering need for expression and to love and be loved. Slowly, my courage and self-awareness began to take hold.

I have grown to love the weights even more, the feel of metal in my hand, the push of my muscles against the force of gravity, the hardness under my skin, the solidity that has helped stop the leaks, given me definite borders. I was afraid I might get bored doing the same exercises. But I have found that within repetition, variety is infinite. Even when I try to make uniform, cookie-cutter reps, they change and spark new creations. I also enjoy returning to the basics as if returning to the same mountain, day after day, with a fresh eye and a different view.

Of course, I have to take time off from training to refresh my body and mind. I also need to break free from a confining schedule and the four walls of a gym, put on my headphones and dance/run/play in the hills, head for the water, stretch or just rest. But mostly, I'm consistent with weight training because I enjoy it. It's my meditation time, my long-term investment for a life full of motion, and it helps keep off some of the fat, sags and wrinkles that wrap ever harder on my door.

I thought my need for motion might fade with time or disappear as I got older, when I was more satisfied in other areas of my life or less capable of full-out movement. But in fact it gets more important and more precious. As I steer into the wide ocean of middle age, it lets me continue to honor that original spark at the core of who I am.

The main difference now is I have more respect for pain. Little injuries or inabilities teach me to work with more intelligence, around discomfort or *with* it, not against the river's flow. This gets more important as I don't want to do anything now that will limit my movement in the future.

In the past I used movement to look a certain way, feel a certain high, grab my life before it escaped me. Now I use it not so much for the extremes but for the steady pleasure it brings. Sometimes I wonder what would happen if I could no longer move. I hope I never find out. But, if I do, I hope I'll still be able to mine the subtle joys of whatever movements I have left. Thoughts like these make me appreciate even more the gift of motion.

I enjoy my strength and the by-products it allows me: to carry heavier grocery bags and make fewer trips, to hoist myself onto a low flying trapeze for an aerial dance class, to climb a rock or a tree. In the weight room these days, I'm actually learning to do more with less: shorter workouts, fewer sets, fewer days a week and the results are actually better than when I trained more often. Maybe someday I'll evolve to the point where I'll simply meditate on movement and that will be enough. But then, when I think about all that I'd miss, I doubt I'll ever let it go.

What Is Strength?

STRENGTH IS NOT simply brute. It can't always be measured in foot pounds or watts. Sometimes it is immeasurable, even invisible. Silence, patience and focus are forms of strength; so are effort, intensity and the ability to confront pain and sit with it. Strength is also seen in whimsy, expansion without fear, a large capacity for pleasure, an angry word withheld, compassion, a smile at an adversary, laughter relieving tension, the eye of a hurricane, a flower growing out of rock.

Strength is not just victory, but the ability to fail with integrity and take the lessons of losing and weakness as opportunities to learn. Like love and wisdom, strength can never be bought or borrowed. Like the earth, it can never be owned but it can be lived in and cultivated. To keep it we must be constantly engaged in the search for it. When we think we've found it and need look no more, we are weakened immediately. And if we use it to bring harm against another in a show of force, then we are not truly expressing strength but power *over*—which earns us a cheap win, passing glory. There's no victory in that because it brings no knowledge. Such power fades after the rounds are fired. Strength, however, when it is slowly, carefully constructed, with failure and frustration as part of the soup, can endure as legend, even beyond our lifetimes.

Such strength comes only with patience, application and honest self-assessment. True strength, by its very definition, cannot come quickly. Overnight strength is simply a mirage—no drugs, money or fame can get it for us, only seeking.

For strength to last, it must come in natural rhythm and its purpose must be linked to something greater than just a passing wish or a trophy for the ego. When it is hitched to a dream others can share, it gathers momentum and grows. Each of us already owns a piece of it. It grows stronger when we offer it freely in exchange. Living in strength gives us no need to wear armor, but the courage to reveal ourselves as we are.

Fear of Strength

"One day a woman that I know came face to face with heroic beauty, that highest beauty which Blake says changes least from youth to age, a beauty which has been fading out of the arts, since that decadence we call progress set voluptuous beauty in its place."

WILLIAM BUTLER YEATS:
"And Fair, Fierce Women"
from The Celtic Twilight,
Dublin, 1893

TO SAY, "I don't want muscles" is no different from saying, "I don't want blood, skin or bone." When we say that, we deny ourselves the right to own something that's already ours. Muscle isn't gender-specific like testicles or ovaries. It's simply the clay that shapes us, fills us all the way out to our edges, keeps us warm, holds us together, lets us move! We lather our skin with lotions; why not indulge our muscles with the type of motion that makes them strong?

Our fear of sprouting big, manly muscles is simply irrational. There's a screw loose in the reasoning process when in one breath we say, "I'd better stick with light weights so I don't get big muscles" and in the next yearn for a body that's "leaner and more toned." Such contradictions reveal a simple lack of knowledge at the root of what we think. No doubt many businesses and manufacturers would like to keep us ignorant, so we'll continue to buy hopes in the form of magic creams, powders and useless exercise equipment. Knowing the truth gives us power to make changes on our own—and to consume wisely. But in the world of female fitness, the truth can be hard to find. There's not even any across-the-board agreement about what a fit woman actually looks like.

On one side of the spectrum, some magazines show skinny models demonstrating exercises with very light weights—too light to stimulate change in most muscle groups. Many writers even *fuel* this fear of strength with statements such as, "Use 1 to 2 lb. weights for 12 to 15 repetitions. Avoid heavy weights so you don't bulk up." Statements such as this mislead and add to the confusion.

First of all, each person's strength is different. Thus, to say which weight and how many reps to use for any given exercise is too general—and can't work for everybody. How do *they* know how much we can do?

Second, the terms "light" and "heavy" are relative to each person, muscle, exercise and speed of the movement. "Heavy" doesn't simply mean anything over 10 pounds. Two hundred pounds can be light on a leg press—even for a not very strong woman. It's all relative. A mixture of both "heavy" and "light" works best.

Third, this word "tone" is just a less intimidating term for "strengthen" or "build." A truly "toned" muscle gets that way by using a blend of weights, reps and techniques that come straight from body-*building*.

Finally, getting "bulky" only happens to a tiny percentage of women who 1) tend to have shorter, stockier builds and shorter muscles, 2) have a higher than normal amount of testosterone, which is genetically predetermined—and occurs in perhaps 1 in 100 women, 3) do lots of power moves such as squats and deadlifts and 4) take steroids. The word "bulky" refers more to body shape than size. Even when a woman takes steroids, she doesn't necessarily get bulky, unless she's already some-what bulky to begin with. But she definitely gets bigger.

Such "big" or "bulky," heavily muscled women pictured in body-building magazines represent the other extreme. They're the ones who get the most publicity as embodying "women of strength." But this isn't reality, either. Many of these women would not have their significant muscle size if it weren't for the male hormones they inject. This isn't female strength boiled down to its essence. It's male strength, in drag.

Instead of striking a heroic point for women, these chemically treated female bodybuilders have actually set back the image of true feminine strength, and in the process have scared away women from weight training in droves. A woman in search of strength and balance need only take one peek at those physiques—and hear an inkling of what it takes to look that way—to say, "If that's strength or health, I don't want any part of it." It's hard to argue that point.

Sadly, the subculture of bodybuilding, especially competitive bodybuilding (amateur and pro), overflows with obsessive behavior, so much so that many athletes, both men and women, have actually become victims of the sport. It's not just the anabolic steroids that create this—but dieting to such unhealthy extremes that it creates eating disorders that weren't there before, or taking diuretics (one pro bodybuilder reportedly collapsed and died from taking these). Add to these behaviors a whole array of pre-contest craziness, including wearing rubber suits and riding a stationary bike in the sauna (to "drop" water); restricting water intake by measuring urine and replacing it with half the amount of water; lowering carbohydrate intake to below 50 grams a day during "carb depletion" cycles, which affects brain function and can damage the liver and kidneys, meanwhile sucking down high doses of supplements (so the body is simultaneously starved and gorged); painting skin with dye used on corpses—and whatever else it takes to please judges, win trophies and get spreads in magazines. For women, the preparation gets even stranger. Since breast size shrinks as body fat disappears, many women feel compelled to get breast implants—also hair extensions, press-on nails, bleach jobs, full-body wax—and with brows, jaws and even genitals enlarged from steroid use, the result is a sometimes Frankensteinian transformation of the original.

Since the whim of the judges for women's contests changes from year to year, even contest to contest, a female competitor isn't sure what she needs to "get it right" to win the title. One time big is in; the next, small, "ripped" and "feminine." So the competitors balloon up or diet down to match the fashion, often getting it wrong and thus creating one more elusive, impossible standard—and one more way to please or fail. So these contests that show women—and men—as strong and powerful really have them going to great extremes to get attention—not exactly the stuff of liberation. All this for what? Glory? Self-satisfaction? The prize money often isn't big enough to justify it. In fact, in amateur shows, competitors often *pay* lots of money to get ready for a contest—for trainers, choreographers, supplements, drugs, posing suits, music mixers, you name it. I don't hear many athletes standing up for their right to be healthy, balanced and drug-free. I don't hear many women in the sport saying, "We're not going to take your stinking hormones" to the powers that judge and take photographs. The pros can't afford to do it because they'd lose their image, their contracts, their sponsors, their income. If there's any hope for rebellion to occur in the sport, it may have to happen on the amateur level.

Personally, I think the whole notion of physique competition is too results-oriented, anyway. Its focus on the finished product reflects the shallow side of our culture. I'd rather see an emphasis on the process. I like to watch athletes *training*, to learn from their form, their method, how their personality is reflected in their approach. A physique contest ought to include actual weight lifting, with athletes doing dueling sets of, say, a bench press—not to see who can lift more but to judge style, finesse, the ability to lift without cheating, tempos, body position, the little half-reps or holds, even the looks on their faces, the sounds they make or withhold. It's in these moments when an observer can see what an athlete is made of and the focus it takes to be a champion—either on a posing dais or in one's life. Bodybuilding contests highlight the elusive results that often disappear just days or weeks after a show. Focusing on process would switch the emphasis to the methods of strength building that endure.

Those of us who train not for a contest, but for life, have to chart a different course. With no competition date in sight, we train for a different reason—for goals that are more far-reaching and less obvious. Although competition can be a great teacher (despite the high levels of obsession), training for solidity in oneself requires a different type of endurance. We have no choice but to weave strength as a tapestry, one layer at a time. Without the jump-start of drugs, our muscles don't show up right away and our strength grows slowly, somewhat like our sexuality. We may start in low gear but once we get rolling, we can go a long way and surprise ourselves with our capacity.

Still, so many of us fear our physical power and shy away from developing our muscles. Why, despite evidence to the contrary, is it still such a ticklish subject, such a frightening path? I sometimes wonder if we're afraid of anything real, or just lazy and in search of a giant excuse.

Or is it much deeper than that? Could it be that we fear becoming too attractive or too powerful?

Women who were once obese and have lost a lot of weight often claim that when they look in the mirror, they still see themselves as fat. In this same way, many of us still see ourselves as weak and dependent, even if on the outside we're self-made and secure. So many times I've heard women yearn to be strong and lean and make a plan to get that way then let something, anything knock them off course. Why does this happen so often? Could it be we have an unconscious belief that if we're strong, we might not be rescued? If it looks as if we're stronger than that man over there, will he be afraid to ask us out to dinner? If we show too much capability, perhaps others won't see our *vulnerability* and will assume we don't need anyone to love (not true, of course). Perhaps some of us associate being strong with ending up alone.

If we've always associated love with protection, then if we appear strong, who will love us? Yet when we're weak in spirit, we're more likely to fall into obsessive, dependent relationships—not mutually supportive ones. Of course, it's possible to be strong in body and weak emotionally—and weak in body and strong emotionally. But when we are weak in both body and heart, we're more likely to look for rescue and confuse it with love, because in times of desperation, it's hard to see the truth. Yet when we set about to find the strength within ourselves first, whether in our bodies, emotions or both, then we can love from a place of strength and fulfillment—as a choice, rather than a need. This way we increase our chances of creating an equal partnership, not to mention the fact that in a gym or health club, we increase our chances of finding someone on a similar, healthy path. I met my husband in a gym.

Physical strength helps during times of weak emotional strength because it is tangible, measurable, and there to return to on bleak days when our doubts run high. Physical strength also informs the heart and mind how to handle a rough situation. If we can sit with the discomfort of a weight on our chest, we can also learn to sit with the times of desperation, loneliness, crises. If we throw the weights away just as we get slightly uncomfortable, how does this mirror our behavior in other aspects of life, when times get tough? Here, we can actually see our behavior and learn not to whine, kick and scream, look away, make excuses. We can transfer some of those same methods to dealing with the petty insults that occur in our lives and the great challenges to our health when we're tested to the core.

One of the greatest lessons about weight lifting is the relationship with failure. I can think of no other place where failure is success, where the desired outcome is to go until we truly can't go anymore. If taught well, we're encouraged to march right up to the wall of failure, confront it, sit with it and absorb the sensation. We get to observe ourselves—either how we dance around in rebellion or are silent, sit still and fail with "integrity intact." When we learn to be unafraid this way, we alter our definition of failure, welcome it rather than fear or avoid it, make it part of the ingredients of success.

Growth often signals big changes—and change, even good change, can be tough to handle. When the change is about expansion, evolution, becoming who we imagined ourselves to be, a foundation of strength gives us a history to draw upon. If we've taken three years to bench press our weight, we can take those same methods of progress and apply them to handling a big change—a little bit at a time, with an occasional big leap forward. Sometimes it means growing beyond jobs, relationships, living situations—even digging into the dregs of our bank accounts or our belief in ourselves and starting all over again. That's never easy. But the daily confrontation with our fluctuating levels of strength mirrors and informs how we handle the big changes in our lives.

I believe that on an unconscious level, this fear of strength has been programmed into us for hundreds of years and is part of a collective memory many of us are just waking up to. For centuries, weakness has provided a valuable survival tactic for women. It has let us hide out during times when those in power sought to destroy everything intuitive, earth-based and feminine. No doubt if we had developed our muscles or our speed during, for instance, the time of the Inquisition or the Salem trials, we would have been branded as born-again Amazons, hauled away as witches and burned at the stake. We would have been regarded as possessing powers that didn't belong to us, male powers, godly powers—and in the male mind, we would have to have been destroyed. Any obvious strength or ability would have threatened our position as subservient females. We had to find *invisible* sources of strength back then—intelligence, faith, fantasies and secret societies. In some parts of the world, this tactic is still essential. In countries such as India where murdering women is barely regarded as a crime, a physically powerful woman might easily turn the weapon on her assailant, upset the whole structure of the society—or require even bigger weapons to bring her down. No wonder, then, that physically powerful women are still afraid to come out.

But in today's Western world, the majority of women no longer need the shield of weakness, though many of us cling to it. It is my hope that if we begin the evolution here and show it can be achieved, it will reverberate around the globe.

We can speak all we want about self-esteem and empowerment, but unless we "walk the talk" how will our daughters and granddaughters know what we're talking about? Do we really need to pass on our negative obsessions with our thighs that keep us numb, afraid, dependent? The more we know how to handle those thighs—and not scorn them in the process—the freer we are from the self-inflicted choke hold they have on our mental and physical health.

The first steps always begin with what we think, what we want and how we plan to follow through. Each of us may need to create our own definition of feminine power. We may also need to grant ourselves permission to be beautiful, sensual and strong. Look, the prison door is open. If we so desire, we can become that towering woman we may have fantasized about when we were kids. There's no one in our way—and there are plenty of others watching our every move, waiting for inspiration, permission and their chance to do the same.

In the more than ten years that I've been training myself, other women and men, I've noticed various patterns of behavior. Each gender has its frailties and advantages, not just physically, but psychologically, which to me is much more profound since it reflects our thought processes, the very core of our characters. Some could argue that these behaviors come programmed in our genetic code. I don't think so. I think they are learned and therefore can be re-learned or, better yet, blended into a whole that pulls the best from each gender.

Women tend to be better learners. We take a humble approach and usually aren't concerned if we look awkward or weak. We're much more likely than men to ask "where am I supposed to feel this?" or "am I doing it right?" We possess a more natural tendency to feel out a movement for ourselves and therefore move more slowly. Men, on the other hand, often lift much faster and have a more goal-oriented approach. If they're reaching for 10 reps, by God, they'll complete 10, no matter how horrendous the form. They have a greater tendency to lift not from the muscles but the ego. It takes a man who is extremely confident in his method to reach not for the heaviest thing he can lift, but for an appropriate weight, even the lightest weight, one that will let his motion be full and his form be true, especially if there's another man nearby, hurling around heavy iron.

Men could use some of our humble, intuitive, cautious approach. But we could borrow more of their "mighty warrior" method. We tend to be much *too* cautious and limply use the same little 3 lb. weights for years and years, never challenging ourselves. We may justify this by saying we're afraid that heavier weights will make us big or cause injury. But more often than not, this is an excuse not to work harder, simply to stay within the same comfortable parameters.

Women and men also seem to have a different relationship to pain. Some men seem to actually *like* pain. Getting into a bar brawl or playing football without padding bring a satisfaction most women can't comprehend. We get enough pain in our emotions, in childbirth and in so many of our relationships. Why would we seek out more? We endure with weight training not when we focus on its pains but its pleasures: the pleasure of motion or the joy of our own company.

Beneath the veil of gender, each *person* has his or her own unique set of abilities to cultivate and shortcomings to overcome that we bring both to the weight room and to life in general. Under this light, we are really all the same, each doing our best with the tools we've got. We all wake up under the same sun, feel the same effects of gravity and time, must answer to our own codes of self-responsibility. Weight training used to be a men's game. Now there are more women doing it. No matter how weak or strong we are, we're all testing and extending the limits of that strength and occasionally flirting with the far reaches of pain. This makes weight training a unique arena where both women and men can meet on more even footing than perhaps we ever have before.

Something has been stirring in the group mind of women. We're reaching out for something—something even beyond equality—back to a knowing, a power that belongs to *us*. These roots are deep and old and have always been there, but we're just seeing them again for the first time. Some don't want to see or aren't ready yet. But those who do see them are forming small collectives, groups, even religions. The earth is peppered with strong women—some obviously so, some not. We circle the globe like satellites. Our searching extends beyond the body to our mind, our bank accounts, our souls, even to other dimensions. We can sense things—other people's thoughts and feelings, when the phone is going to ring and who it'll be, how events are going to turn out, how time seems to bend, how there is a grander scope of justice that weighs out all actions, thoughts and words. It's not necessarily "psychic" ability. It's just an ability. We may even sense that our bodies don't end with our skin— but expand beyond to other etheric bodies as well that some of us have the power to see and heal. Many of us may not see this with our own eyes but, from instinct, know this is true. Our knowledge of those worlds, of the forces that run both the macro and the micro cosmos we live in, begins in what we see, hear, smell, taste and touch. We learn the ropes on the physical plane, but it doesn't end there. No doubt we can train ourselves through meditation or some other sort of practice to feel the various subtle energies that flow through us and into others. What better place to begin than in our bodies? Are they not the vessels of our souls?

Our muscles certainly aren't everything—just part of the whole picture, but a part we can choose to develop if we long to develop as many parts of ourselves as we make time for. The purpose of getting strong is to embrace more of life. The ironic thing is, as we wake up in our bodies and in our minds, we become more aware that any minute we can die. Yet, as we become more alive, the fear of death diminishes. It no longer hangs there as the dark, ominous henchman, ready to snatch the lives we haven't fully lived (or even started), but becomes something different— a light, another option, a journey home. If we open ourselves to the sensations of being alive, the pain, the rejoicing, the pulse of this magnificent force that trumpets through us every moment of the day, then we can say that we lived, we experienced and perhaps did the things we came here to do, sipping from even the seemingly insignificant moments in life, full sensation, all emotions, including high amounts of joy.

The Sensuality of Strength

What is it like to dwell in a strong woman's body? How does it feel to have muscle coursing down our limbs, like tresses of hair tumbling down our backs? What's it like to house a marriage of opposite forces within one body—the soft and hard, active and yielding?

It is running through a forest, like Diana, goddess of the hunt, with a slim-hipped powerful engine rolling the hips and lifting nimble feet over rocks.

It is the independence of carrying two suitcases down an airport corridor—finding competence in the sheer weight of them, with no "poor little me" in sight.

It is the intersection of a hard pectoral meeting the soft handful of a breast, and the gristly sinew of leg muscle entwined with the putty of a thigh.

It's knowing how to pull up in the head, neck and chest, and down into the pelvis—to be able to fly in one moment, and in the next, sink legs down like roots of a tree.

Our power grows from the earth, feeds on iron, air, heat, food, love and water and travels through a lifetime. We cannot trace its source back to a true beginning or see where it will end.

We are in fact the vessels of new souls—and we carry them into life. But we also carry others with us as well, chosen partners and ourselves on other loving journeys. We are at home in dream time—and can bring our dreams to reality. Every one of us has special powers. We are dancers on the edge of infinity.

Why We Need Strength

GETTING STRONG because we "should" isn't a good enough reason. "Should" stirs up guilt, obligation, getting serious, buckling down. It's our mother's tone of voice, our father's lifted eyebrow—the look that needs no words but says, "Get in here right now young lady. Just what do you think you're doing?" "Should" cracks the whip at our back, is hidden beneath every self-criticism and resolution, runs counter to every craving, pits the taskmaster against the devil.

Some people thrive on "should." Rigid personality types who like routine, clear boundaries and restrictions, find it's a turn-on because it structures their world. More carefree personalities tend to be oblivious to the concept, order another bottle of wine, eat the whole box of chocolates, buy lavish gifts for friends. "Should" hardly enters into the vocabulary—but it probably "should" more often.

It's nice to know that when we're motivated to get stronger "because it's good for us," our time is wisely spent. But let's not suck the joy right out of it, just because we "should."

- Strong muscles help us stay lean. Muscle is "active" tissue (unlike fat, which just sits there, making sure we don't starve during long winters and are always "plump" enough for pregnancy). With more muscle in our bodies, we use up more calories even just sitting around; our energy needs increase, so our metabolisms speed up. It's as if our engines now idle at higher r.p.m.'s. We have to eat more, more often. Sometimes the hardest part is getting used to the idea that eating more is okay and won't make us fat, as long as the meals are low fat and relatively small. (If we eat more than we can metabolize at one time, the extra is stored as fat, even if it's nonfat food.) Being hungry more often is a good sign that our metabolic fires are lit and working more efficiently.

- An average weight training session uses about 300 to 500 calories an hour—depending on intensity. An average aerobic session may use the same. But a study at the University of Oregon (by Goldberg and Eliot) showed that weight trainers used about one-third more calories than the aerobic exercisers did, *after* the session was over.

- Muscle weighs more than fat. So when a person drops fat, adds muscle and depends on the scale for feedback, she might not recognize progress. A body fat test, the way clothes fit and the overall tightness of muscles are better indications of results.

- Building muscle is more than an appearance issue. It also decreases our risk of contracting health problems associated with high levels of body fat, such as heart disease (the #1 killer among women, according to the American Heart Association), diabetes and cancer.

- Dieting without exercising wreaks havoc on our body's ability to shed fat. After deprivation, our bodies, in their desire to seek balance, come off diets fatter than before. The poor little fat cells hold onto everything they can. The want us to live—not starve and die.

- Aerobics require muscle *endurance*, rather than strength. The movements make us sweat and build up some strength in the related areas (runners have strong legs, swimmers strong upper bodies, and so forth). But they don't offer the deep cellular stimulation available, for instance, in a set of deep squats or a bench press. Exercises such as these make our muscles adapt to the loads we give them, and therefore, after a workout, they go into a recovery period (typically lasting two days) in which our muscle tissues repair themselves and come back stronger. This doesn't happen so much with aerobics. Bodies that do aerobics only may shed fat—but the muscles don't always tighten up; body shape doesn't always improve.

When muscles get stronger, they grow into a more pleasing shape, as if realizing their potential.

- Stronger muscles improve problem areas in posture—especially protruding abdominals/weak lower back, sunken chest/weak upper back. When these areas are strong, we stand up taller, and also reduce our risk of winding up with "dowager's humps" on our little old lady backs—making us easy prey for muggers and purse snatchers!

- Training eases misalignments and muscle imbalances. "Pear-shaped" women, for instance, with slightly knocked knees, hip and ankle pain, can correct some of the problems by strengthening their quadriceps and hamstrings—especially if they also do impact motion such as walking or running.

- Upper body strength lets us carry our own weight in the world. It literally "arms" us to lift our children, carry heavy suitcases, haul pieces of lumber. It also decreases the typical 35% gap in strength between the sexes (though we have only 20% less muscle mass than men)—and helps erase the concept of women as the "weaker" sex.

- Training appears to "slow down" the aging process. Unused muscles shrink about 10% with each decade. Weakened muscles also make it much less fun to move. So naturally, activity decreases and metabolism drops, while body fat, aches and injuries sky rocket. Growing old then becomes a real drag. People think we get fat and out of shape because we get old. No, we get old because we get fat and out of shape.

- We can get face lifts, collagen injections, breast implants, calf implants, and even have eyeliner, eyebrows and lip color tattooed on our faces—but not one plastic surgeon in the world can inject us with all-over, naturally built, vital-looking muscle! Muscle is the cheapest beauty aid around. Contrary to what many believe, muscles don't reach a certain age and say "OK, that's it. I'm no longer going to react to any outside stimuli." Over time, our muscles can continue indefinitely to get both stronger and more defined, although they won't, thanks to our female hormones, get much bigger.

- Muscle strength adds density to our bones and reduces our risk of osteoporosis. Bones need "weight bearing" exercise to encourage the production of more bone cells and calcium. Other factors besides weight bearing exercise, however, help prevent osteoporosis. It's also important to:
  - Get sufficient calcium in the diet
  - Make sure exercise isn't *excessive*, causing a body that's too lean—which disrupts periods (and inspires eating disorders).
  - Pay *extra* attention to exercise and proper nutrition when we go through menopause because the drop in estrogen needed to maintain bone tissue decreases the bone's ability to create calcium.

- Walking and running are weight bearing, but only for the lower body—where many of us are already strong. We need all-over strength. (Note: It's a bad idea to wear wrist or ankle weights while walking or running, in an attempt to add "progressive overload" or add an upper body workout. These can throw off alignment and put an unnatural load on the joints. Weights and fast motion don't mix.)

- Water exercisers need to add land-based training to their regular water workouts. Although water resistance strengthens, heals and rejuvenates it doesn't have that big G for gravity, which aging bones need.

Strength training and other types of exercise in general also help:

- Relieve stress

- Improve endurance, reduce fatigue

- Lower blood pressure

- Ease symptoms of PMS (although some days that's hard to believe), reduce cramps and length of menstrual cycle

- Promote lower levels of total cholesterol—with more of the good kind and less of the bad, thus preventing heart disease

- Possibly prevent cancer

- Improve self-image and self-esteem

- Provide greater mental focusing skills

- Heighten the sensitivity to our bodies' needs

- Give us greater peace of mind and ability to relax.

The Journey In

"Make haste slowly."

BENJAMIN FRANKLIN:
Poor Richard's Almanac

WHENEVER I HEAR someone say "I really *should* get in shape," I know it's a safe bet they won't. Guilt is a terrible motivator and it's no fun. But when someone says "I *want* to get in shape," the outlook is bright. Guilt isn't powerful enough to fuel a long-term commitment, but desire is.

Vanity's a surprisingly good motivator. It kicks us off the couch. But it can't sustain us for very long, either—even vain people get bored. In time, vain actions feel empty; so we leave them in search of others with more meaning.

We have to go deeper if we want to stay in this game for a while—seek out food for the mind, touch into the heart and soul. The problem is, the route to those deeper places isn't a straight, easy shot. We often find various bits of wreckage strewn along the way—mental weakness, whole areas of physical neglect, even heartbreaks, and negative self-images. If we can just keep in mind that the intended outcome of this search and cultivation of our strength is to come out on the other side, strong, healthy and striving toward inner peace, then the journey makes sense. If it's all struggle and outward appearance, forget it. The mission is to go in there and bring ourselves out in all our glory. This prize, like all things of great value, doesn't come without some tests.

This is true for both men and women. I believe we all carry the blueprints of our lives in our muscles, joints, organs and the way we move. But women, in particular, hold shame in dark, hidden areas of our bodies that we pinch, scrutinize and judge in private. The chest stores our sadness and low self-worth, and our pelvis is loaded with sexual history and vulnerability. Traumatic experiences get wedged there—sensations of having been battered, silenced, abandoned, abused, unloved, unattractive and unappreciated. Out of proportion to reality, we often then see ourselves as fat, ugly and misshapen—not just in our bodies, but in our experience as well.

This vast cavern of despair we feel about our bodies has driven us to great extremes. We've certainly made many people rich, trying to correct what we see as our defects: We'll go on liquid fasts for months at a time, have our jaws wired shut, our stomachs stapled to half their original size. We'll binge and vomit, get the fat sucked out of our thighs and transplanted to our breasts and pay thousands of dollars for every sort of reshaping a plastic surgeon can do. But none of these radical "solutions" addresses the core issues of what created those feelings of despair in the first place, and how we can counter them on our own. Not one of these things inspires our imagination, reinforces our belief in ourselves or gives us practical tools of change, based on our own abilities. I have nothing against money, doctors or even plastic surgery. But these are better used only after cheaper, homegrown, intuitively guided, common-sense methods (like exercise and a balanced life) have been exhausted.

From my own experience, I've come to believe that negative obsession on certain parts of our bodies actually freezes energy there. If we hate our thighs, wear baggy clothes to hide them, go on butt-breaking regimes, then measure the changes every day, we actually slow up the process. Our focus is misplaced. Demanding change doesn't work. It's more effective if we focus on the work and let the changes take care of themselves. Transformation is not simply a matter of the will; it has its own natural pace. Forcing it or checking it too often is like trying to make a plant grow faster.

Therefore, we need some faith to get through various "black nights of the soul" when we see no results but must keep going regardless.

We also need courage. As body parts start to wake up, we may encounter some strong emotions and deep issues—some not so easy to deal with. Strange memories might come flooding in. (I have cried on a leg press, screamed out on a horizontal squat machine—masking my emotional pain in perfectly acceptable gym groans and grunts.) The more we're willing to allow them, the sooner they'll pass—and the sooner we'll see results. This is almost like a "breaking in" process, like breaking a wild horse, but gentler. For instance, to work the buttocks muscles effectively, we have to "get down" into deep, open positions that can make us feel very exposed. Some of these muscles may have forgotten how to flex or surrender. As we become more articulate with them, other parts of our beings seem to come alive as well, including the shadows. As much as possible, it helps to resensitize these areas with patience and compassion.

Forcing is traumatic for both the body and spirit. Any rapid change in the setting of the weight room is to be avoided. Trying to do too much too soon, we hurt ourselves, get sick or burned out and thus give ourselves no choice but to back off for a while. "Falling off the horse" this way really isn't so bad as long as we get back on. It's a form of self-preservation, a wise message from the body and the imagination to "find another way."

Slowing Down

In the beginning of a strength-training program, it's not uncommon to double, triple, even quadruple muscle strength in just the first few months. After that, progress slows down to a more natural and common pace—poco a poco, bit by bit.

Our bodies get strong in layers. At the very beginning blood flow increases, skin tightens, muscles harden under the skin. Later, tendons get stronger and more elastic and bones acquire a new density. This process is fairly simple, quite linear and takes months to a few years.

The initiation of the mind, however, is more complex. Depending on the individual, the ability to focus can be immediate or take a lifetime. And because our mental state is always shifting, this aspect of training constantly changes. Progress here isn't linear at all. The path loops, spirals, spins back on itself and occasionally seems to dead-end. Sometimes we get pulled off course completely. But, with practice, it takes less time to come back.

Novices should begin training slowly, with long, full repetitions, to get a true feel for or command of the muscle. This brings more muscle fibers into play but also heightens focus, builds awareness. Three questions should dominate this process:

- Where do I feel it?

- Where am I *supposed* to feel it?

- How can I improve my form so it feels right?

When confused, tired, frazzled, weak or in a hurry—slow down.

This is good medicine on many levels. I don't know about you, but as a modern woman, I often suffer from hurry disease. I've been known to suck down black-sludge cups of caffeine, speed down the freeway while eating lunch, shop like a contestant in "Supermarket Sweep," make twenty phone calls in a row and forget who I'm calling, say, "Yes, I can do that" to everyone who asks a favor, "multitask" with four open windows on my computer at any one time, speed through an aerobic workout to a pulsating 140 beats per minute, zap dinner in the microwave, while tossing a salad, while putting away the clean dishes, while talking on the phone and cleaning up as I go, then later cruise through the channels to find something to numb me or hold my attention. Whew! I've even gotten a charge out of the frenzy, because I can actually *pull it off!* But I can't help but wonder, what do I get for all that? Where am I going in such a hurry?

Strangely enough, the place where I slow my r.p.m.'s is in training—and this, I believe, is why I've stayed hooked. With weights balanced at the ends of my limbs, I have to slow down, feel, think. The stakes are too high if I don't. If I get careless or rush, I could hurt myself. And I can't just cruise through on autopilot, either. I've got to show up completely. Over the years, I've learned that I get my best results when I take a moment before I start training to "ground" and stretch. Then I pick up weights with care, keep check on my form throughout and afterwards take a moment to appreciate the work I've just done, rather than judging myself for doing a bad job or rushing into the next thing. This has sparked a major breakthrough.

Now, as much as possible, I try to apply this approach to other activities in my life—waking up, cooking, eating, driving, writing, making love and unwinding before I go to sleep. My seemingly meaningless activities have become more sacred and rewarding and consequently, I'm calmer, healthier, nicer to people. Although these little periods of "nothing" are silent and invisible, they've become even more valuable to me than the actions they frame. Without them, I'm caught off balance, once again swept up in the hack job of my life, and feel angry, rushed, shortchanged. But with these silent pauses, I seem to paint a colorful inner world. Inspiration comes, and the magic starts to work.

The Principle of the Iron

RESISTANCE IS a fact of life. Drive any rush hour, dress a screaming baby, talk to an irate customer and we deal with resistance. How we react to it shows the world and ourselves a part of who we are—and sometimes it's not a pretty sight. We may hate the feeling—but none of us can escape the way it seeks to permeate our days and irritate our weak spots.

To be weak against a force increases the risk of being overpowered, injured. To be rigid against it makes us vulnerable to being knocked over, getting our bodies and egos snapped in two. However, when we learn to absorb, deflect and redirect the resistance to our advantage, we come out in balance.

At the center of resistance work is discomfort—one reason why so many avoid it. The discomfort needn't be extreme or prolonged. But it's necessary to train ourselves to stay in it, if only for a moment, because this is the moment of both conflict and opportunity. As we move into the hard part of an exercise (or situation), we are literally transported to a more condensed state of being where time and sensation expand. What we do next is key. Do we fight, scream and throw the weights down, rushing to get it over with? Or do we slow down a bit, expand our sensation, breathe into it, hold it for a moment and quietly finish? It doesn't take a lot of muscle to pull this off. It takes the mind. And a little class.

The principle of the iron is simple. It is not just what we do, but *how* we do it, that determines the outcome. The iron itself is passive, inert. *We* bring the life to it. We supply the motion, power, intelligence and creativity. We add the mood that makes love with the weights or battles them. We bring the mind that makes ten pounds feel like a hundred or fifty feel like five.

The principle of the iron is always in action. What we end up with is the sum total of our method. In other words, when we train with struggle and rage, what we get is more struggle and rage. When we train with impatience and sloppy form, the result is more impatience and sloppiness, which leaves us unsatisfied and possibly injured. Yet if we train to learn something, build strength and experience more pleasure, we end up stronger, wiser in many ways, exuding an air of delight.

In Balance:
Hard and Soft

IN A FAST AND VICIOUS WORLD, seeking balance within ourselves seems the only road to sanity. Out of balance, we spill the coffee, back our cars into walls we don't see, run the race of our days a step or two behind. In balance, we shift into low gear as the world rushes by, drive with an eye open to obstacles and create time to enjoy the scenery.

The very definition of balance as "a cancellation of all forces by equal or opposite forces" means we need to meet the rushing tides with just the right amount of internal push or flow. Otherwise these forces flatten us or we flatten them. There isn't one ultimate way to be that defines "in balance." External and internal circumstances are always changing. That's the challenge of it. The search for the center point constantly shifts. If we are too hard, aggressive and quick, something usually snaps. We alienate people, hurt ourselves and often sit alone in anger. If we are too soft, we become pliant in others' hands, feel invisible, get taken for granted.

Many women have sought the hard, active, yang forces in order to survive in a "man's world," keeping all hints of weakness far away from work. But it's tough to wear that mask all the time. We fatigue; the strain takes a toll.

Many of us have also cultivated the soft, inward yin forces that find us happy puttering in the garden, reclining in the bath, curling up in a window seat and looking out at the world. Yet, despite the peace we feel doing these things, we might feel guilty whenever we hear those driving voices say, "Go out there and *do* something." By itself, receptivity doesn't seem to do enough to justify its existence in a "go-get-'em world."

When one mode dominates our lives, we lack the resiliency to meet an oncoming force and/or flow with it. By itself, just the yin or yang makes the circle only half complete.

This same concept of balance applies to exercise as well. Our bodies like it both ways—hard and soft. But too many of us hook into one form of exercise because it's easier to follow a routine. Performing just one sort of activity is like eating one type of food. We don't get enough different nutrients.

To find balance in exercise, we ought to seek out hard and soft styles, either in an array of exercise choices or in the subtleties within any *one* type of exercise. At first glance, some types of exercise appear to be only "hard" or "soft." Yet, looked at closely, each is a full world unto itself and contains a bit of both.

Weight training, for example, is obviously "hard." It hardens the body and it sometimes feels "hard" to do. Yet for the body to harden and truly "absorb the weight" it must have moments in which it is soft and receptive, not fighting. There needs to be a surrender within each repetition, a stretch at the "bottom" of a movement, a moment of stillness for gathering forces, so we can do the hard part of the motion in a way that's strong but not rigid.

Running is also "hard" in that it jars our bones. Yet we can soften it by changing the surface, running on dirt or sand. We can soften the impact if we vary strides—run backwards, add a skip, move side to side, add little bitty steps, blend it with a walk.

Swimming might look soft because the water is yielding. But depending on how we use the water determines whether the activity is hard or soft. When we move languorously it's all softness and surrender. But when we churn the water, press and pull our way through it, we hit up against its density, confront its hard wall.

Tai chi, a "soft" style of movement, may look to some as if it does nothing, takes no effort at all. Yet to acquire a grounded solidity, the "rooted" tai chi stance requires that we sink down into our legs in a way that is anything but soft. Tai chi masters can throw people across a room with a "soft" sort of power that is practically invisible.

A similar thing occurs with yoga, also traditionally "soft." From the outside, there may appear to be no movement, nothing happening except static poses. Yet inside, fires burn as we struggle to surrender our stiffness and free our breath.

When we look at all our activities this way, we begin to see a blending of forces and can start to ask ourselves various questions:

- What sorts of exercise do I normally favor—hard or soft?

- What do I need to add for balance—more hard or more soft?

- Can I explore the not-so-obvious hard or soft side of my favorite activities?

- What am I in the mood for today?

If we're feeling soft, a soft sort of exercise may or may not be the right choice. We may need the energy of a hard style to "get things moving" and create balance by going to the opposite. Or perhaps, when we feel especially vulnerable, our wisest choice would be more softness, to complement our mood. Each situation is different. When we ask what we need and check in with our "wiser selves," the answer usually becomes apparent.

If we choose all softness, we have less energy, since the demand isn't so great. When we overdo hard motion, especially as we get older, we know it for the next few days. It's as if there's a cosmic accountant out there tallying up our scores, noting that when we take too much from here, we lose a little over there. We *feel* these laws of cause and effect.

In Balance with the Elements

Another way to find balance with exercise is to look to the example of nature—the grand master of equilibrium. In ancient myths, astrology and works of art, the four elements have always symbolized balance. With four elements, the balance is even more solid than with just two (think of a four-legged chair, as opposed to one supported by just two broad legs). The picture is bigger, the landscape more complete. One or more of these elements is present in most every dynamic, transformational occurrence on our planet. Since we are mini-worlds as well, it's natural to look to nature as a guide to our own wholeness.

Our bodies also take on the quality of the element we favor. If we only go to water, we become a bit "watery." If we choose only iron, our bodies harden like armor. A blending of elements give us a more complete balance. But it's also important to note that each activity might have a dominant element and a smaller degree of other elements in it as well. For instance, wind surfing is an air-based activity, but water obviously must be present, and lifting the sail requires a bit of strength work—an earth-based action. Thus there is a mini-balance of elements within the sport. It's interesting to note what elements we favor, and to see if one is obviously missing. By seeking to blend all four elements, we may discover one we had forgotten and truly love.

Some questions can help in this search:

- What element is most obviously present in the type of exercise I do most?

- Is there a balance of elements within that activity?

- What element do I love the most?

- Is any element missing?

EARTH

The earth is home, the great role model and master of rhythms. It never stops moving, changing, renewing itself, and yet its cycles are consistent and predictable within a given range. The Chinese refer to this as the Tao or the way. The way is change. The earth, seemingly, doesn't resist this change. Yet how often do we humans fear it, clinging like cats to a tree, even when change is for the better?

The earth shows us how change works at different intensities. Slow change evolves. Children grow; seasons unfold. Sudden change brings catastrophe—floods, earthquakes, raging fires. These are natural rhythms, too. But when the earth swings out of balance it seeks whatever way it can to right itself once again, regardless of what's in its path.

Tremendous wells of energy are stored in the bowels of the earth— oil, gas, minerals—immeasurable riches. On its surface is beauty, paradise. Almost every one of its landscapes is a masterpiece of precision, order, magnificence, except those scarred by human invasion. It's delicate and hardy, too. We are its watch-keepers and its destroyers, depending on what we do. We serve the same function with ourselves.

The element of earth offers us an abundance of opportunities for improving our health. We can hike its hillsides, dig our hands in its soil, scale its rock faces, even just lie on a grassy field and let the earth work its healing power. Outside, cradled in the wide open belly of nature, our doors of perception fly open. We see things in a new way, are "grounded" once again.

When we lift weights, we literally apply iron, an element that forms in the earth, directly to our flesh. The weights are dense and comply with the earth's laws of gravity. We must be grounded, centered and aware to work with them correctly. The body even craves the sensation of iron, just as it craves the mineral iron when it is anemic. There is a primal, carnivorous kind of appetite for it as the weights literally "arouse" our muscles into greater awareness. Once touched by iron, we too, become solid as earth.

WATER

We began our lives in watery wombs, floating in warm, wet sacks. Our flesh is 90% water. We need a constant rush of fluids to flush our systems and keep us alive. Without water, our cells could not squirt nutrients. All energy production would shut down, and flesh would shrivel off the bone like wax paper.

Throughout our lives, we bathe sorrows in tears, rinse away soiled memories, wash those loves right out of our hair. Water lets us start again new. A spring rain coaxes life out of rocky soil. A tide pool is the seat of creation. A warm bath is salvation on cold winter nights.

Water does not discriminate. It seeks all openings, sits level above bumpy places. If we fight it, it takes us under. Yet, if we play with it, it lifts us up. In its arms, we are graceful again, light as elves. And when we learn to use it wisely, make circular currents with the flick of a fin, spin eddies off a cupped hand or the flash of our mermaid's tail, we paint, sculpt and dance with it. We are at the center of our own creation. It scrubs our spirits clean.

We may meet the water horizontally, vertically, in the shallow, on the surface or in its depths. Yet whatever way we choose, we enter it and like nowhere else, are instantly transformed. The water takes gravity and neuters it, pulls the rug of friction out from under our feet and forces us to shed all regular laws of motion that apply on land. Getting from here to there challenges us to think. As swimmers, we need to streamline our bodies, cut away all unnecessary drag. As water walkers/runners/exercisers we must hit the water upright, using every way we can to maximize the resistance all around. Our goal isn't speed but to generate as much resistive force as possible. In its soft, nonforcing way, water works its power into the trenches of our deepest, hard-to-reach muscles—if we know how to use it wisely and not jump around in it, but meet it with sensitive, spiraling limbs.

As water yogi/ballerinas, at long last, we can take our legs up to *there* and feel all the grace we may have only dreamed about. Miracles are so common here, they often go unnoticed.

FIRE

Fire is the flashiest of the elements. It can erupt almost out of nowhere and lick its yellow tongue over everything in its path. It can enfold a house, a hillside, a whole city in a matter of minutes and push its way wherever there is fuel, air, a place to move. Fire can be Lucifer's agent, leaving nothing but charred remains, ashes, coals. And it can also be the angel of warmth, home fires, cooked foods. Fire is the transformer, takes matter and alters it, often destroys but sometimes purifies and, like the alchemist, turns base metal into gold. Like the other elements, it either supports life or ends it, depending on how we meet its power and if we know how to use it wisely.

The godchild of fire is movement. Fuel turns to heat in a series of sparks, combustion and explosions, powering cars, rocket ships, bodies. Without fire there would be no propulsion. Without heat there would be stasis, ice and no animal life at all.

To build a fire to last, we must light it slowly, especially when we've grown cold from inactivity. If we light it too fast, it flames for a brilliant minute and dies. But when we coax that ember glow with patience, blow on the flames and add timber as we need it, the heat grows steady and engines purr. Fire can then go to work, turning tension into motion and melting fat for fuel.

Sometimes when we light the fire of aerobics, we also start too fast, flare up and then burn out. Yet when we build the fire slowly, the cauldron burns at a steady pace. It radiates not only from the heart, but from the core, and sends a cleansing steam coursing down our limbs and out our pores. What works best is a low, slow, red and white heat. Glowing embers. The warm bath of sweat seems to melt stubborn old bits of sludge, sets out the garbage that accumulates within. Dancing in the fire, something wild is set free. An occasional flame may rise up to lick the inside walls—a hard interval, a steep hill, a hot sun overhead. But to keep from burning up, we have to monitor that heat, keep watch, or we'll literally cook ourselves from within—and it can take two days to recover. Our fires must be put out with care as well, lowering the flame before blowing it out.

AIR

Air is the element we cannot see. We look right through it as if it didn't exist. What we see is its *effect* on other objects—floating dust particles, wind whipping up a cyclone of dirt. It's the substance that supports the fog and clouds, makes space between the raindrops. But the air remains invisible, though it makes its way through our lungs, blood vessels and every cavernous opening in our bodies. It sustains plant life and even penetrates the water and sustains the creatures that live there as well.

Air has form, weight and offers resistance when we drive headlong into the wind. To overcome our own weight and fly an aircraft, we need the power to lift. Once airborne, we can fight the invisible giant of a headwind and wind shear, or we can merrily catch a tailwind and gain altitude, riding a thermal. Yet if we float through space, where there is no air at all, and therefore no resistance, we can orbit toward infinity.

To lift our own bodies into the air, we meet the practical joke of gravity. Anyone who has ever tried a gymnast's flip, a trapeze artist's swings, a dancer's leap—all of which mimic the effortless, airborne grace of birds—knows the amount of energy required, especially to make it look effortless. To maximize momentum and overcome inertia, if only for a precious long moment, takes much preparation and a knowing touch. We have to feel the exact moment that's right for takeoff. Lifting too soon or too late means falling, flight aborted. And sloppy landings mean a crash.

Not too many of us work our bodies directly in air as leaping dancers, gymnasts or aerial artists. Few of us even get to wind surf or hang glide, both of which teach us about currents and moving with the forces. What we all work with, however, is the invisible. Each of us must contend with emotions that seem to ride in on the air, with their own powerful currents and resistance. We all experience busy, noisy, ongoing action in our minds and could use a cleansing breeze.

We seek the air for focusing the mind and honing back to our hearts. The gifts of air aren't obvious or visible. We're in air-based motion when we concentrate on the stretch that occurs *inside* the yoga pose or the simple action in tai chi of shifting weight from one foot to the other. We're in air as dancers, reaching for that frozen moment when we hang suspended, defying the pull of gravity. We're in air in the playground when we swing all the way up—"whee"—and all the way back—"whoa!" We're in air when we first learn how to wind surf and hold still, waiting to catch the wind. We're in air when concentrating on any move requiring precision. And we're in air, with a chest full of sadness or lungs bursting with excitement, when we move through the world, without saying a word.

Part Two
The Mechanics

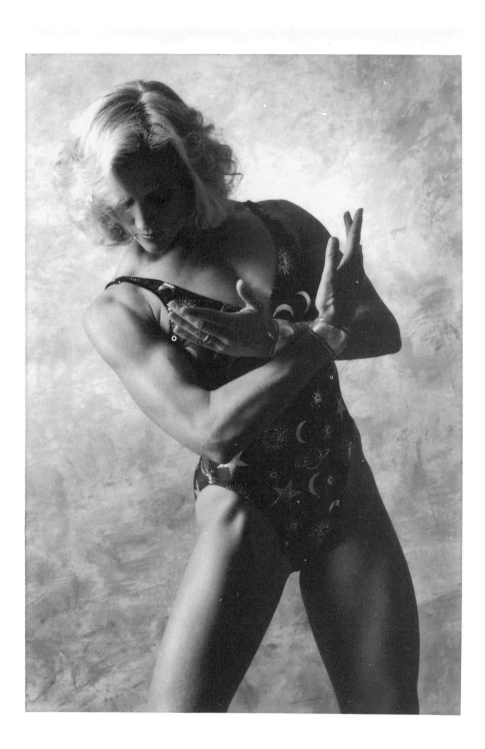

Transformation Begins in Posture

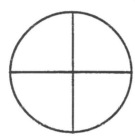

THE WAY YOU HOLD your body broadcasts how you feel about yourself, whether you want anyone to know or not. Posture is the "body language" that dares speak the truth you do not. It says things that perhaps you don't even know.

Most people have some problems with posture, especially as youthful elasticity fades. Habit, time, wear and tear and various traumas can combine forces to create glitches in the way you move and hold yourself upright. The little unconscious actions you perform—always carrying a bag on one side, slouching, cradling a phone in your neck, leaning into one hip, help carve out posture, individual as a thumbprint. Emotions leave their mark, as well—creating sunken, heartbroken chests, the world on your shoulders, chin jutting forward to bite an attacker, rigidly stubborn locked knees, "I give up" big bellies and bowed lower backs. Left unattended, these postural abnormalities can grow into big distortions that impair movement and leave you prone to injury. The odd thing is, you can end up this way and not even know it! Distorted feels normal because you adapt to it. You might not even realize how much energy you put out to maintain it. You simply keep adapting—until one day something snaps, pulls or you can't move without hurting.

Sometimes, after healing emotionally, some of these weak, numb or armored postures drop away. Simply by working on the inside you can learn to "open up" on the outside and carry your body with pride. But the external pressures are always present, especially if you sit all day, work at a job that requires repetitive actions or simply stop moving vigorously. As you get older, the need for good posture becomes even more critical so you can avoid the stiff, hunched-over, shrunken posture of old age.

Some types of exercise can make posture worse, particularly when there's forceful impact involved (as in running, power lifting or heavy contact sports) or when you favor one side, as in tennis and golf. Resistance training done carelessly can wreck posture, too. The combination of bad form, heavy weight and workouts that ignore whole muscle groups can seriously damage discs and joints, limit range of motion and create imbalanced posture. But done well, training can improve posture like nothing else. It can also repair damage earned from other activities—or from no activity at all.

The Weight Training Posture

Almost every sport has its own posture. Tennis is crouched and "ready." Ballet is pulled up. Biking and skiing demand leaning forward, while tai chi requests that you "sink down." The weight training posture is good posture—exaggerated to an extreme. It's not rigid or militaristic but a proud stance that screams to the world, "I feel good," whether you really do or not—though it's amazing how holding yourself like this can clear a bad mood or ease a depression.

In order to lift weights, get results and not hurt yourself, you've got to keep this erect, "open" position *at all times* while lifting, or you can't lift safely and won't be able to fully control muscle contraction in the back, chest, shoulders, arms or legs—virtually everywhere! As effort increases, form tends to fall apart. Thus, the first thing to correct should always be posture.

The Body's Core

The torso is the body's command-control center, the core. When the core is strong, back and abdominal muscles can hold you in a steady, supported position, no matter what the arms and legs are doing—with no hunches, arches, twists or strains caused by the motion. Often, these stabilizing muscles get stronger just from holding up the torso during training. But if you don't have that core strength to begin with, then the first bit of focus should go here. Trying to shape arms and legs on a weak center is like building a house on no foundation. These exercises address those unsexy, unglamorous muscles—essential for developing true strength.

Core Stabilizing Exercises

1. For abdominals. Lie on your back with your knees bent, feet lightly touching the floor (as if your feet are floating on a cushion of air). Gently lift one leg at a time, trying not to arch or "pelvic tilt" (flatten) your spine. Alternate lifting your feet, keeping one foot "floating." (To make this more challenging, take your arms overhead and reach the opposite arm toward the lifting knee.)

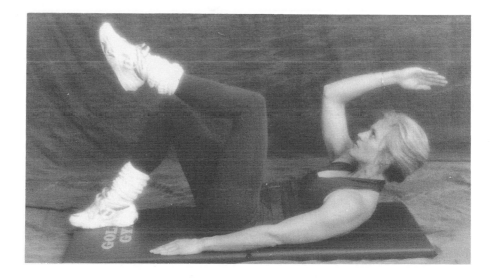

For Abdominals

2. For lower back. Support your body on hands and knees. Raise the opposite arm and leg in a horizontal line. Keep your torso steady, so the hips don't shift to the side. Alternate.

Do 2 to 3 sets of 10–15 repetitions each, every other day. If your core muscles are particularly weak, begin with just these exercises for at least two weeks. Later add them to a regular training program, at the *end* of a workout (not at the beginning—so tired stabilizers don't "poop out" during the workout).

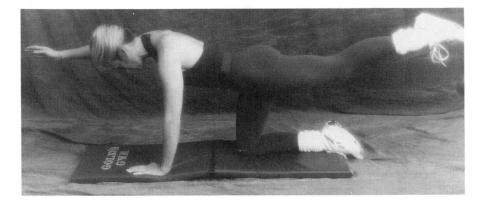

The Posture

Neutral Spine

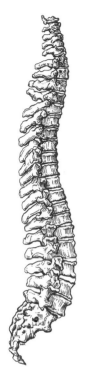

To protect the spine while lifting, it's important to maintain what's called "neutral spine," or the natural S curve of the backbone seen in profile. To keep this healthy "S," *slightly* contract your lower back muscles—don't flatten your lower spine. There should be a *small* arch in the lower back and an opposite arch in the chest as well—so the chest feels lifted and "proud," almost excessively. In this position, you can safely do all kinds of movements—even bend forward. It's like wearing a natural girdle and brace for back and shoulders.

You may have been schooled against arching the back at all—so being told to arch even a *little* might make you worry. Arching excessively is definitely a bad idea—it compresses discs, and you lose abdominal support. But it's safer than flattening (pelvic tilting) or rounding the lower back. Rounding the lower back is the most common mistake I see—and the way most people hurt themselves. When the lower back is rounded or even flat, the back muscles stretch—so lower back support virtually disappears. A stretched muscle can't also simultaneously contract. This dangerous position leaves back muscles and discs vulnerable—especially when you're leaning forward, doing an exercise like a bent-forward, one-arm row.

It's far safer to keep the spine in "neutral." To find the "neutral spine" position, first slump, then carefully arch the back. From there, find the "middle zone." Your torso should feel lifted, supported, ready. This is the posture that works for training. The real trick is keeping it throughout every exercise!

Posture Details

To chisel in the fine points of perfect training posture, start from the ground and work up.

1. Ground and center. Take a solid stance, with your feet about hip width apart. Turn your feet out slightly if that's more comfortable. Feel the weight equally dispersed through the heel, the center of the foot, the metatarsal. Slightly "soften" your knees and gently let

your weight "sink down." This motion should be almost invisible. It's an energy exercise rather than an actual movement.

2. Maintain a strong core and neutral spine by contracting your abdominal and lower back muscles, keeping the natural curve of the spine (as above).

3. Keep your shoulders down and back. Since approximately fourteen muscles attach at the shoulders (back, chest, biceps, triceps, for example) it's important to "quiet" the shoulders so upper body muscles can work effectively. Because of all this interaction (like a maze

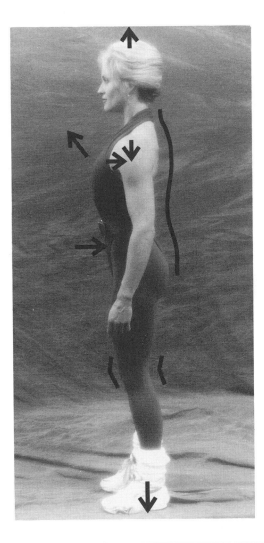

For Lower Back

of exits and on-ramps in the L.A. freeway system), shoulders often jump in to help even when you don't need them. Putting them down and back gets them "out of the way." Shoulders are very quick to shrug or roll forward—and in general are vulnerable to injury—especially any time a bar is pulled or pressed behind the head (a position I generally avoid). Try to keep your shoulders down and back, even when you are working on them.

4. Keep your chest "lifted" and open. When chest muscles collapse, like the back, they can't simultaneously contract. A sunken posture renders chest work useless. This also pulls your shoulders forward, throws off alignment and transfers much of the workload to the front part of the shoulders and triceps.

5. Keep your joints soft. Locking or snapping your joints stresses the tendons and often diverts work *away* from the targeted muscles. It also gives you a false sense of ability when you snap into locked "resting" positions. It's better to work with continuous tension on the muscle (for example, on a bench press or leg press, avoid "locking out" elbows or knees). Instead, keep joints slightly bent even at the top of the lift and, instead of letting muscles rest, put the mind into "hardening" them.

6. Beware of "breaking" the wrists, the weakest link in the chain of arm joints. People with weak wrists might consider wearing wrist cuffs both as a support and a reminder to keep them straight (especially for those who work at a keyboard all day or others at risk of getting carpal tunnel syndrome, a painful wrist condition caused by overuse of that part of the body).

7. Keep your neck in line with your spine. Tuck your chin slightly down and in, as if "opening a window" in the back of the neck. Pull up your head as if it dangles from a string.

Align the Body in a Cross

If all of the above is too cerebral, detailed and tough to remember, the following simplifies alignment beyond words. You can maintain balance by sensing a constant connection between the vertical and horizontal lines of the body. This helps the posture stay true and improves placement.

The Vertical Line

The dominant posture line is vertical. This infinite line runs down from the sky, through the center of the head, through the spine, out the tailbone and down into the ground—or it goes the other way, starts in the earth and travels upwards. Whatever way one visualizes it, this is the body's axis, the center line, the active, "masculine" yang force. By extending this imaginary line beyond the body, you can better "anchor" yourself further into the ground, so you don't lose balance—and it also helps you project energy up. This serves as a reminder that physical energy doesn't end at the boundary of the body.

Every time you round forward, arch or twist the spine, stick out your chin or sink your chest, you break the vertical line. To heighten awareness of this line, it helps to stare at an existing vertical—a pole or a seam in a wall and align with *it*—or "step into" the vertical, as if stepping into a ray of sun, a cylindrical shaft with narrow walls, that limits all movements off the axis. This vertical line works even when you're horizontal or inclined forward on an oblique.

The Horizontals

The horizontal lines are smaller, more subtle. Actually, you have many horizontals. The major ones are the neck, shoulders, hips, knees and placement of the feet. Any time you tilt your head sideways, lift one shoulder, favor one hip, bend one knee, or put one foot too far in front of the other, you break the horizontal lines. The horizontals require balance. When something goes wrong with posture, the subtle horizontals are usually affected first. They represent the receptive, reactive force, "feminine" and yielding. The horizontals and the vertical should stay at a clean 90-degree angle to one another at all times.

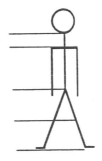

The "Whole" Body

In bodybuilding terminology, the body is often referred to in sections: quads, pecs, lats, delts, and so forth. This sometimes gives the impression that you're just a group of muscles that never quite blend into a whole. This isn't so. Ironically, working muscles in small detail lets you develop more precision and "total body awareness" than if you worked your body as a whole. There's more of you at your command. The landscape is richer. Eventually those details tie together and tell a story of a self-realized body, one that has been lovingly molded, reworked, retrained.

During this process, a new type of self-awareness takes root. You begin to sense how alignment is disturbed just by the shift of one hip. At first, you may not always know when placement is wrong—or, when it is, how to correct it. But when it's right, the vertebrae stack on top of each other like nesting dinner plates, and energy flows. Movements come unimpeded and everything suddenly falls into place. When you tune your senses to the fine art of body placement you not only determine whether or not the exercises will be effective—you determine the very essence of your well-being. Then the message that radiates from your posture becomes one of pleasure and glowing health—a reflection of the healing process that takes place both inside and out.

Intelligent Use of the Forces

Gravity

Strength training is a game of gravity. What you're working against is the steady, downward, unchanging sheer magnetism of objects being pulled to earth. Simply put, your job is to lift a weight against that force and then control it on the way down so it doesn't fall. Sounds easy . . .

Three Types of Lifts

Type 1. When you work with free weights, you work against a simple line of force. You lift the weights up; they want to fall down. What you're resisting against is the pull of the weights to the *floor*, the direct line of gravity—straight down. Although this sounds logical, I often see people failing to take this into consideration. An intelligent use of this force, for example, is a flat dumbbell flye (photo 4), in which you lift the weights directly on the gravity line.

A not so intelligent use of gravity would be performing that same flye while seated upright in a chair (photo 5). Although the intention might be to work the chest, the downward pull of gravity exerts a far greater workload in the *shoulder* joints and muscles, which in this exercise are supposed to be only secondary. Here, the chest doesn't receive the full benefit of gravity, doesn't get a good workout and the shoulders end up stressed.

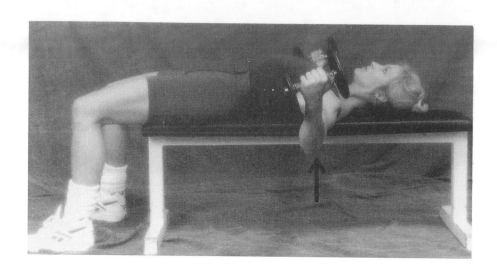

Intelligent Use of Gravity

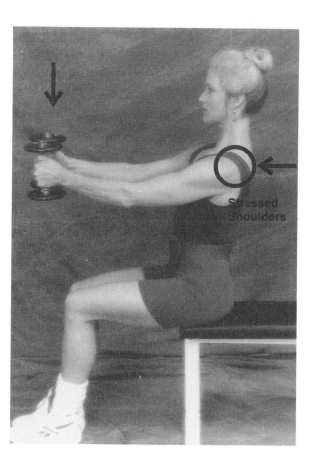

Stressed Shoulders

Not so Intelligent; "Stressed Shoulders"

Type 2. Any time you work a machine, you add one more element. Whenever there's a fixed point, such as a lever arm or an overhead or floor pulley, you pull or push against *it*. Of course, gravity is still in effect pulling things to earth, but the machine should be designed so that you don't just fight the downward pull, as you do with free weights. You've got a "fixed point" and you push, pull or curl directly against *it*. What you need to know is how to position your body in relation to that point. Subtle changes affect different areas. For example, on a seated cable ₁ow, when the pulley comes from above, the lower back and lats do much of the work. When the cable is directly in front, it's the mid-back and lats. When it's low, it's the upper back and lats. You can pretty much draw a straight line from the fixed point to the working muscles.

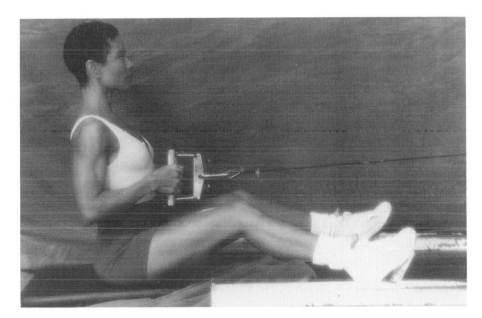

Pull directly against a fixed point.

Type 3. Then there are lifts or motions in which gravity plays a smaller role. When you work with resistance bands, for instance, you can do movements that wouldn't work with free weights because the bands are light and gravity doesn't drag them down (only the weight of your limbs does).

In fact, astronauts on the Space Shuttle used Type 3 lifts when they worked out with Dyna-bands (a type of resistance band) in gravity-free outer space. They didn't need gravity to create resistance (though they did need their strengthening exercises, since in space, the lack of weight bearing down on bones causes bones to decalcify at a rapid rate). Strengthening moves in the water are also type 3 lifts. Here again, because gravity is minimized, you can work muscles on all sorts of angles, without a thought about gravity's downward pull exerting force on the joints. In water, the resistance is all around, making the water like one big, 3-D weight machine.

Type 3 lifts, especially with resistance bands, often work best when combined with a fixed point—as in Type 2. In other words, it's best to pull in *one* direction with a band—and a fixed point helps accomplish that. Pulling in two directions at once—for instance, down and apart (as in a two-arm lat pull down with a Dyna-band)—breaks the line of force in two, and thus disperses the resistance. A smarter way to do this exercise is with one arm at a time, holding the other arm over your head in a fixed point.

Regardless of the type of lift you do, the general rule of thumb is that whenever you perform a resistance exercise, the point where you make contact with the resistance should end up either directly *over* (as in a bench press), *under* (a one-arm dumbbell row), *in front* of (front raises for shoulder) or *across* from (lateral raises) the muscles you're trying to work. In other words, there should be an obvious, clean connection between the resistant object and the muscles in question.

Every Joint Is a Pulley

The body is both very smart and very lazy. Give it a job to do, and it will recruit as many muscles and joints as it can to get the job done. Its objective is to spare energy. But the objective with weight training obviously isn't to make the job easier but harder, more localized. Thus, you've got to *outsmart* your body by focusing the work only in the area you intend. This means only using the joints you really need.

Muscles are like ropes and joints the pulleys that lift your bones. Any time you use more joints, it's like using more pulleys. You get more "leverage advantage." Whenever you do an exercise, you should use only the necessary joints to get the job done. Because the body is smart and lazy, other joints will take over—unless you consciously keep them still.

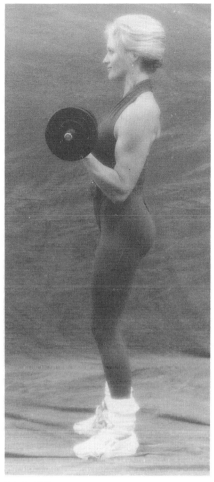

Right Way—
"One-Joint Move"

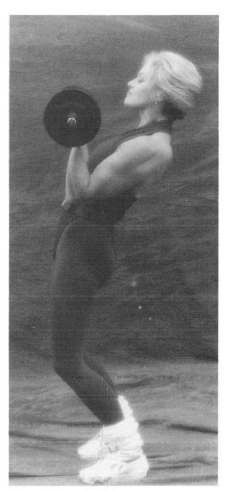

Wrong Way—"9 Joints
Activated"

Look how many joints want to jump in to assist a nice simple, one-joint exercise, such as the biceps curl:

1. ankles wobble (activating foot and shin muscles)

2. knees bend (activating quads)

3. hips thrust forward (stretching hip flexors and contracting buttocks)

4. lower back arches (making back muscles contract)

5. shoulders shrug or roll forward (lifting trapezius muscles)

6. elbows lift forward (activating front shoulder muscles)

7. wrists bend (using forearm and hand muscles)

8. chin sticks out (tensing neck muscles)

9. thumbs wrap around bar (one more leverage advantage in the grip)

That's nine ways that work gets diverted *away* from the biceps, since each joint will yank on its surrounding muscles to a certain degree. Each joint may divert only one to ten percent of the force. But when you add it all up, that leaves very little true work for the biceps.

The Underlying Geometry

There's a simple geometry that unites all resistance exercises. It's so simple, in fact, it might seem obvious. Yet that's the beauty of it. When you use it, shapes emerge, patterns are revealed. For instance, there's consistency to all pressing motions, similarity among all pulls, curls and flyes. Seeing these connections helps you apply the same rules to all similar motions, rather than exploring them one by one.

To see what I mean, imagine the weights are actually paintbrushes that trace the path of motion. Every repetition "marks the air" with either a straight line or a circular arc. No wobbly lines, ovals or ellipses. Every strengthening motion in its purest form boils down to pure lines and arcs. Learning to "draw" these shapes on the outside helps you better "see" on the inside. (Later, if you want to add a slight turn of the wrist here, a twist of a limb there, that's fine. Since muscles often attach on a diagonal, you may find you get a better "final squeeze" by adding these little punctuating motions in some exercises. But it helps to understand pure movement before you build upon it.)

Lines

Moves that use two or more joints, such as presses, squats, pulls and lunges, draw straight lines. In other words, the path of greatest resistance is straight. These lines can be vertical, horizontal, oblique, parallel or intersecting—and can meet at a point or cross at the midline. Whatever the angle, they need to be *straight*.

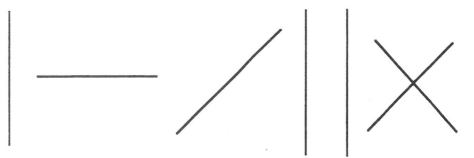

This line is "the line of force" or straight pathway of resistance as it travels through your body. It's easy to *see* on someone else when it breaks and goes wrong. For instance, in a regular free bar squat, the clean line of force should travel up through the heels, hips and shoulders (photo 8—right way). At the bottom of the squat, the torso inclines

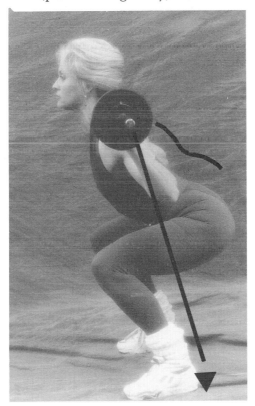

Squat—Right Way

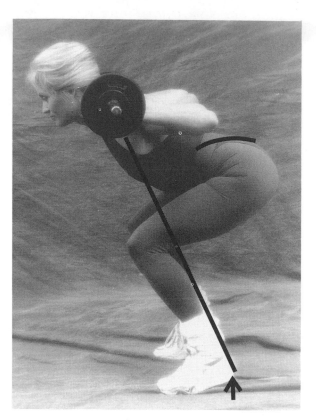

Squat—Wrong Way

forward slightly, so these joints stack up just off a vertical line. As you straighten your legs, you return to a vertical line.

However, if the torso dips too far forward as you lower, the line bends—and the bulk of the load gets transferred into the lower back (photo 9—wrong way). If the heels lift off the floor, some of that load then transfers to the knees. By bringing the shoulders back and the heels down, you keep the line clean.

In a stationary lunge, the line is vertical and matches the spine. In fact, the main weight that's been lifted here is the torso, whether or not any handheld weights are used (photo 10—right way). The "line of force" travels up through the back of the knee, hip, spine and shoulders.

If the torso rounds forward, arches, or wobbles from side to side, the weight gets unevenly distributed and the clean line is broken (photo 11—wrong way).

You can't always see the "line of force" as it travels through your body,

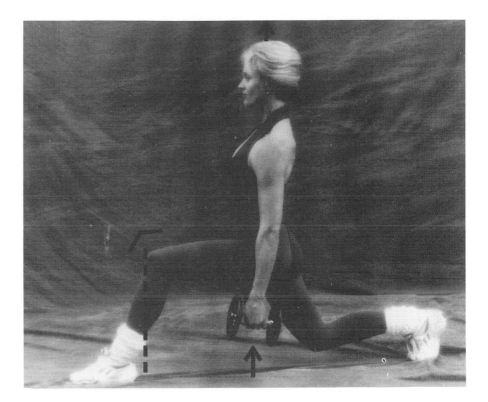

Lunge—Right Way

since mirrors aren't always strategically placed. However, by keeping watch over the *angle* of the joints, you can see when a particular muscle group is getting used or overstressed. For instance, when a knee bends more than 45 degrees, particularly when it's combined with a forward motion (as in a step-forward lunge) it literally *points* to that area taking all the punishment—the knee. Shorten the knee angle to 45 degrees, and that knee no longer absorbs so much force—the force gets dispersed to working muscles. Or remove the step-forward action and do the lunge in place, and the forward force is diminished.

Multi-joint moves that "draw" straight lines are also called "compound exercises" since they use more muscles. More joints give you greater leverage advantage—so you can handle more weight with these exercises. Such motions form the foundation of both beginner and advanced programs and are especially valuable for building strength and power.

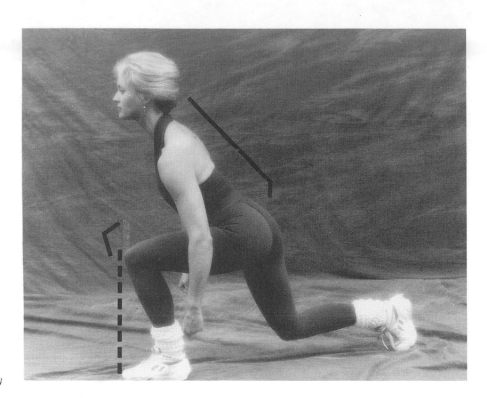

Lunge—Wrong Way

Arcs

One-joint moves such as flyes, curls and leg lifts use arcing motions. These arcs can be quarter circles, half circles or somewhere in between. Arcing motions imitate a compass, pivoting around a fixed spot. Wherever you hold the weight, cable or band traces the *perimeter* or outside of that circle. At the *center* of that circle, or the sharp fixed point of the compass, is the single moving joint. The muscles that initiate this movement are the ones being worked. In other words, every time you do a one-joint move, you're essentially "drawing" the shape of a rainbow. The muscles that initiate the movement can be found at the center of that circle, like the proverbial pot of gold.

By shifting the position of an arc, you shift the muscles that do the most work. For instance, a flye is a basic one-joint move. Depending on your body position, you can do flyes for chest, medial delts (mid shoulder muscle), posterior delts (rear shoulder muscles) or lats. But a flye is

a flye is a flye, and the rules are the same for each—keep elbows soft and trace the *outside* of a healthy, round circle.

Arcing motions localize the work into a specific area and are also called "isolation" exercises. Therefore, with these exercises you should use less weight. They're valuable for strengthening, sculpting and fine tuning.

Using the hours on a clock face can help guide you through the proper range of motion for each arcing exercise. Let hands or feet point out different "hours" on the clock. Think of the top of the head as 12 o'clock for most of the exercises, to help place the body in space.

Which Comes First: Compounds or Isolations?

All workouts, therefore, essentially consist of multi- and one-joint moves. It helps to think of them this way when planning workouts. The question then comes up—when to do what? That depends . . .

Doing the straight-line, compound or multi-joint motions first lets you use up stored energy in powerful motions. When you want to "go for it" with heavier weight, do these first. An example of this would be doing leg presses, squats and/or lunges before leg extensions or hamstring curls—bench presses before flyes.

However, on days when there isn't such an abundance of energy, it makes sense to "pre-exhaust" muscles with isolation, or one-joint work first. By doing flyes before bench presses or leg extensions and hamstring curls before leg presses, quadriceps and hamstrings come into the multi-joint movements already tired. It takes less weight to fatigue them, so you can get a good workout using less weight.

Levers

If a short person and a tall person of about the same strength capabilities stood side by side doing biceps curls with a 30-pound bar, the shorter person would have an easier time. Why? Because the shorter person has less space through which she needs to drag the weight. Her bones, or levers, are shorter, giving her a leverage advantage—so the weight feels easier to lift. The shorter person usually also has shorter "muscle bellies," which take less time to develop, because there's less space to fill up with muscle. So, chances are the shorter person will get stronger faster, as well.

Shorter people may develop more quickly but sometimes tend toward a stocky build and, thus, should avoid a full diet of heavy weights. They should also add more moderate and light weight exercises, plus aerobics and steady eating habits with low-fat foods—since stocky bodies can easily look plump. Lat work can also help build a "V" taper in the torso, which will create the illusion of a long, narrow waist.

Moderate-limbed people can build physiques that are both powerful and aesthetically pleasing—and can achieve this best with a combination of heavier and light weight training for size, endurance and aesthetics, yet should also supplement training with aerobics and low-fat foods to avoid looking "blocky." They tend to develop muscle at a steady, moderate pace and often have height to lend elegance to their bodies.

Long-limbed people take the longest time to develop. Yet once they do, their bodies look aesthetically very pleasing—a combination of long lines and curves. At first, they need to concentrate on some basic, multi-joint moves like bench and leg presses to build overall functional strength and put "meat" on their bones. Later, they can add more isolation exercises to sculpt specific areas. Long-limbed people should continue aerobics for cardiovascular conditioning and make sure they eat *enough* low-fat food to sustain new muscle growth.

Everyone, despite body types, benefits from a mixed approach—and a balance of cardiovascular conditioning and healthy, low-fat foods. This variety of methods and all-over conditioning better prepares your body for the variety of challenges you face in real life.

What Is Full Range of Motion?

People talk about the importance of "full range of motion" for the muscles and joints, yet I think it needs to be more closely examined. Many assume that big motions must be good because they use more muscles. It's that "more is better" mentality: "If my arm can circle all the way around like this, then if I put a weight in my hand and do it, I work more muscles through a full range of motion movement. And that's what I want, isn't it?" Not necessarily.

Muscles are all intricately attached. Any time you move, you activate a whole host of them. Each muscle has its *own* full range of motion, before passing the job along like a game of hot potato, to yet another muscle. Pure muscle isolation, therefore, is a pie-in-the-sky concept. No muscles act alone. Yet you can better control which *group* of muscles you want to focus on if you simply use the range of motion for that particular muscle group. The challenge is knowing where to start and stop. The exercise section of this book gives these specifics. But once again, using the posture, quieting unnecessary joints and "drawing" the underlying geometry helps you stay within the right parameters.

Avoid the Dead Zone

To get the most out of every repetition, it's wise to avoid staying too long in the "dead zone," where muscles are essentially resting. Examples of this are locking the knees during squats and leg presses, locking the elbows on bench presses, letting the arms curl too high on a barbell curl or, when using bands, letting the resistance slack.

Stopping in the dead zone for a quick breather, to "buy" more energy for better repetitions, is fine every once in a while to enhance the end of a set. But going there unconsciously and between every rep doesn't yield the best results.

Momentum

Power and Olympic-style lifters heave much more weight than bodybuilders—but in many cases, their bodies look blocky, fat, not at all sculpted or defined. Olympic-style lifters especially (who perform such fast-paced moves as "the snatch" and "clean and jerk"), tend to lift with lots of momentum and, in the process, "blow out" their knees, shoulders and backs. What does this tell you? To strengthen and chisel your muscles and extend the life of your joints, avoid using momentum (and too much weight).

Any time you lower a weight, gravity generates momentum. At the "turnaround" point where a lower becomes a lift, you can use momentum to buy yourself a sizable portion of the following lift. It's a bit like rolling through a stop sign. It's harder, yet more "honest," to come to a complete stop.

This way, when you stop for a split second in a stretched position, you let the muscles "absorb" the weight. You just need to be careful not to overstretch when the weights are heavy and when joints feel overtaxed. Lifting "dead" weight is much harder. Yet it's a truer picture of what you can *really* lift, not a quick satisfaction for the ego.

Give Muscles a Full Menu

Your muscles are:

- Strongest when lowering a weight (an "eccentric" contraction) because they get assistance from gravity.

- Second strongest when holding a weight steady (an "isometric" contraction—in which muscles are rigid).

- And weakest when lifting (a "concentric" contraction) because they're working directly against gravity.

Each type of contraction works and fatigues muscle fibers in different ways. In real life, you don't just lift your loads, you also have to hold them for a while and carefully set them down. Thus, you should employ the same combination in your workouts. This shouldn't just be called weight lifting, but weight holding and weight lowering, as well. (For a detailed description of incorporating all three, see "Transcendental Repetitions.")

Reps, Sets, Weight and All That Jazz

Good Pain, Bad Pain

Before venturing boldly into the uncharted territory of a new exercise or training in general, it's wise to use caution—especially when nursing an injury. First, "test the waters" with a half motion or light weight before doing the whole movement or exercise. See how it feels. If it hurts, try it from a different angle, slow down or use a shorter range of motion—but avoid pushing through sore spots. If an exercise still hurts, try a different one. There's no shortage of variations to choose from.

It's important to know when to "tough it out" to expand strength capacity and when to "fold" to avoid injury. Here, pain can be an ally and a guide. There are basically two types of pain involved:

Bad pain tends to:

- flash (like red lights in the brain) saying, "Careful, INJURY"

- be sudden and sharp

- focus in the joint—not the muscle

- occur on one side of the body

- and linger . . .

Good pain, however:

- builds slowly (like heat in a fireplace)

- is dull at first, then prickly

- tends to focus in the belly of the muscle—not the joint

- occurs in both limbs simultaneously (i.e., bilaterally)

- disappears immediately after the exercise is over

- but shows up as muscle soreness 24 to 72 hours after a workout, letting you know the muscles were working.

The Quality of Repetitions

Muscles can't count. They feel. Therefore, form, not the number of repetitions you do per exercise, should be the first concern when learning how to lift. Once you can hold yourself properly through an exercise, *then* the number of reps starts to matter. However, if you can't keep the form, then you don't get much out of the motion—no matter how many reps you do. One good repetition with solid form is worth more than ten fast and sloppy ones—because after one good rep comes two. It's a place to begin.

The first order of business when performing an exercise is opening the connection between the muscles and the mind. This doesn't take special powers—simply a willingness to be quiet and feel, a desire to "be present" to what's happening and concentrate. No matter how weak you think you are, you can enhance the *quality* of each rep, hypnotize and coach yourself with simple words such as "yes," "focus" and "good form." Although you may not "glide over the wall" of discomfort and muscle failure the first few times, you *can* do it early on in training, since this takes *mental* rather than physical strength. As you allow yourself to "come alive" in the discomfort and yes, even "the pain," something inside shakes, roars and wakes up. You might even grow to like it—or at least bask in its afterglow.

How Many Reps?

Different numbers of reps elicit different reactions—yet this also depends on the amount of weight being lifted. In the traditional school of weight training, the rule of thumb is this:

- 1 to 6 reps with heavy weight—build power and increase strength

- 8 to 12 reps with moderate weight—increase muscle size

- 15 to 20 or more reps with light weight—build muscular endurance, but don't necessarily increase either strength or size

When you can do the full number of reps with ease, then, logically, it's time to move up in weight. But this isn't always the answer. Sometimes when you move up in weight, you can only do two good reps—in which case, it's a good idea to do those two reps and finish the set with lighter weight (called a "descending set"). Simply adding reps can be a good choice, too, especially if you don't do high-rep training very often—or if the goal is muscular endurance. So—how do you choose? The answer is to let form be the guide. With good form and focus, you can pull value from all sorts of techniques.

As for the final word on the effect of different reps, researchers are still exploring whether the rep ranges given above do what you think they do. Many bodybuilders claim to get great results using occasional high-rep training—with reps as high as 50 or 100 (one of the most grueling workouts; the lactic acid build-up is almost unbearable. However, many believe the pain is worth it, since it leads to greater muscle hardness and definition). Many more swear by a steady diet of 20 to 30 reps for leg exercises since leg muscles are big and can endure, while others use the low reps of power lifters to increase strength and size. Whatever research may reveal in the future, a variety of approaches and reps will probably always work best and lead to more balanced development. The different reps and weights also keep the *mind* alive.

Counting

It's not wise to place a self-imposed rep limit on your muscles, which are very suggestible. If you tell them 12 reps, that's all they'll want to do.

Why stop at the obvious "rest areas" anyway? Why do 8, 10, 12 or 15 reps? Why not let the muscles make that decision and stop at 11 reps, 13, 17, 22?

I often "zone out," forget to count and don't worry about the numbers unless I'm trying to do more than the last time or am working one limb at a time and want to be even on both sides. Counting is one, but not the *only*, way to keep the mind engaged. (Sometimes I overhear personal trainers doing nothing more than counting reps, when simple reminders about posture would be more valuable—especially at upwards of $50 an hour!)

Numbers, however, give us something to hold on to, the satisfaction of a goal, a way to measure performance. Rather than counting from 1 to 12 (a long way to go), try counting reps in groups of 3's or 4's, breaking the set into manageable pieces. Or try counting 1, 1, 1. This way there's only one rep—and one more!

How Many Sets?

The number of sets (or groups of repetitions) you need per exercise depends on how effectively you do those sets—and how many other exercises you do for that body part. It also depends on what you're trying to achieve and how much time you've got.

Some people may sufficiently "get inside" a muscle with only one or two sets per exercise. Others need three to five. People who need more than that probably aren't concentrating or working hard enough. Making every rep count cuts down on the need for so many sets. More isn't necessarily better. Doing too many sets can actually produce diminishing returns. It's tough to contract a muscle when it feels like bubble gum with the flavor chewed out!

You've done enough sets when:

- strength significantly dips

- muscles keep shaking well after the exercise

- the muscles can't hold a contraction.

On the other hand, you might not have done *enough* if:

- there's no feeling of muscle fatigue after training. You should feel as if you've "run out of gas," a sign that the body has used up all the glycogen (or carbohydrates) stored in the liver—the energy source for strength training.

- muscles aren't slightly stiff or sore 24 to 72 hours after a workout.

As with reps, the number of sets is variable, and it's best not to get attached to doing the same number of sets—always 1, 2 or 3. The secret to success is being willing to shake up a routine.

Beware of long workouts—the overachiever's demise. After an hour and a half of training, muscles actually start catabolizing—eating themselves for fuel! Forty-five minutes to an hour and fifteen minutes is about perfect for a weight workout. Less is fine, too. I try to limit myself to twenty or thirty minutes per body part—1 to 3 body parts per session.

How Many Exercises?

How many exercises you need to improve or maintain fitness is a personal issue, and one you discover only with time and practice. Needs also change. Larger muscles like the back, chest and quadriceps may need at least three different exercises—especially for development from different angles. Smaller muscles such as arms and calves can probably get away with just two. This also depends on how you divide body parts. Obviously, if you work the whole body in an hour, you don't have time for so many exercises. But if you divide the parts (see "The Splits"), then you've got more time to devote to each—which, in my opinion, is a more thorough method.

Order of Exercises

Start with larger muscles first, so the warmth generated there can radiate out to smaller muscles. For instance, it's not smart to fatigue smaller, assisting muscles, such as shoulders or triceps, and then expect to bench press. The smaller muscles give out first—robbing the chest of its chance to work effectively. A logical order would be chest, shoulders, triceps. Likewise, it makes sense to work the back before the biceps, the quadriceps before the inner thigh, the hamstrings before the calves.

It's also recommended that beginners avoid working abdominal muscles first, since these act as important stabilizers for almost every exercise. If they're fatigued before starting, they might not effectively hold up the torso. Plus, when abdominal exercises are saved for the end, the muscles come in "pre-fatigued" and therefore won't require so much work.

However, I sometimes "break the rule" and do abs first—to make sure I do them! (When I save them till the end, they often get short-changed.)

These rules exist for a good reason—to protect people from getting hurt. But sometimes, in order to make your own discoveries, you have to be adventurous and bend or break the rules—and perhaps find out why the rules exist in the first place. You just have to be responsible enough to handle any consequences—and this comes only over time.

Fast Twitch/Slow Twitch—Muscle Fibers in Action

Each of us is essentially made up of a mixed bag of fiber types. Very simply put, we've got slow, moderate and fast twitch fibers. The slow twitch fibers help us sustain long bouts of aerobic endurance and enable us to walk around and stand up. Moderate twitch fibers help us through extended sessions requiring muscular *endurance*—as opposed to strength. "Toning," for instance, with lots of reps and light weight, is a moderate fiber activity. Fast twitch fibers come into play in short bursts of activity—such as a 50-yard dash or an intense set of biceps curls. Most weight training calls on fast twitch fibers, since most sets are of fairly short duration. Yet all fibers may be recruited to some extent or another, depending on how you train.

Each of us has a different distribution of these fibers. Our bodies also adapt to the workloads we give them. A trained endurance runner, for instance, usually has more slow twitch fibers; a power lifter, more fast twitch. There is some debate about all this—a chicken or egg type theory. Do people with more slow twitch fibers naturally tend to become long distance athletes or do long distance athletes metamorphosize their muscle fibers into slow twitch to achieve their desired ends? No one seems to know for sure.

Weight training is traditionally a fast twitch activity. Yet using different weights and rep speeds can recruit more fibers and perhaps more *types* of fibers as well. A mixed bag of methods once again (both in the weight room and cross training in general) leads to a more complete development of different fiber types. The end result leaves you better prepared to meet the different physical demands presented in life.

Rep Speeds

2 UP, 4 DOWN

This is the basic, safe tempo for traditional weight training—especially good for beginners: 2 seconds to lift and squeeze, 4 to lower (counting "1-1 thousand"). By keeping the negative twice as slow as the lift, the lowering is more controlled, with less assistance from gravity. Over time as you learn more control, you can speed up the negatives to 2 seconds. (In a muscle conditioning class, music with 120 beats per minute works well—with 2 counts up, 2 counts down, using the slower "main" beats as your guide.)

Yet, even with this moderate tempo, the temptation is to rush. The majority of lifters make the mistake of going too fast—doing reps in 1 to 2 seconds. When I go that fast, I spend 60% or more of each rep *resting*. I don't have time to add an extra "squeeze" at the top of the motion, my negatives fall to earth and my next rep rides up on the wave of momentum. It simply becomes a lactic acid wash, a goal reached without much consciousness, a thing to be gotten through, but isn't as "mindful" or intense. Rushing is not only ineffective, it leads to carelessness and injury.

THE 10-SECOND REP

By slowing down to what feels like a crawl, each rep becomes a test of both strength and endurance. Going slow maximizes the time spent in contraction. A solid 10-second rep divides the lift into 4 seconds up, gives 2 full seconds in a "squeeze" and leaves 4 seconds to lower. Working at this tempo takes high concentration and since no momentum is used, it's hard to cheat—thus, less weight is needed.

Although going slow may not suit everybody's nature, it's a good practice to begin with—and to return to often, as it's the truest style of weight training I know. Using this method, I've gotten stronger than when I lifted heavier weights at faster speeds. From time to time, I return to heavy weight to see if my method really gives me the muscle to power through heavy sets. It does. Such slow, patient movement also seems to strengthen the tendons more effectively as well and results in far fewer injuries.

10 DOWN, EXPLODE ON 1

This is perhaps the most intense type of training. Allowing 10 seconds for the negative lets you better control that weight through every inch of its journey, without "sliding" through the tough spots. Once you are in full stretch position, the lift should come in an explosive, but controlled, 1-second motion. In my mind I yell, "fire" or "explode" each time I do this. After only a few reps, the muscles stop obeying my command, become rubbery and dimwitted. The explosive moves fizzle, the negatives melt away in a sticky mess. A good way to finish off a set that's falling apart like this is with moderately slow reps—to regain control of the movement.

This advanced style of lifting seems to call on the slow, moderate and fast twitch fibers all at once—anything to get the job done—and truly leaves the body quivering.

Half-Reps & Holds

Another way to add variety is to explore various sections of the lift. Try adding pulses at the bottom half of the motion (usually the toughest part), followed by pulses in the top half, followed by full range of motion repetitions. (This method is often called "21's" because the traditional method is to do 7 reps of each.) Also, find the sticking point (the toughest part of a lift, where it's no longer possible to continue without cheating) and just hold the weight without sacrificing form. Try counting to ten. This may be the longest 10 seconds of your life, but it makes the isometric a dominant part of the set.

A Good Fail

Taking the muscles to the "absolutely can't do another rep" stage is what's worshipped in bodybuilding as the ultimate victory. "A good fail" is a muscular action, not a mental one. To get there takes training, and is tough at first for beginners. I also believe it isn't necessary to reach this point on every set, despite what others may say. Doing so can be too draining physically and psychologically. It's just one tool in a bag full of methods. Yet, using it can be quite a rush!

To approach muscle failure, first you must navigate mental failure (like sneaking past Grendel in the medieval woods). The mind says, "That's enough. Stop!" But the limbs usually have a few more repetitions in them before failure is true. This is the pain zone, the dark night of the soul for your nerve endings, a test of might, courage and character. As long as no "bad pain" demands your respect, you simply must keep going, like brave and humble knights, onward into the dragon's den, wrapping your chattering mind in a soundproof box, freeing your breath, opening your eyes to the experience and your nerves to the sensation—even if you've had no training for this at all. This is not the time to jump around and scream so others can hear, notice, or rush in to rescue. This is the opportunity to keep sensations private, to still extraneous motion and not sacrifice form just to finish—but fail with integrity intact and, perhaps, just hold the weight as above. Or, if a training partner is present, let her do the lifting while you focus on the lowering. If you can push through failure, you travel deeper down into your own dragon's den where you mine the most precious strength of all. This is where you face yourself, stripped of fear and excuses. This is where you're raw and striving, equal to all others who also take themselves here. This is the work that not only gives substance to your body, but to your character as well.

Though this may sound like self-inflicted torture, the pain here is nothing compared to the emotional dregs or spiritual crises you often have to endure in your outside and inner lives. The pain here teaches you something about the pain there—except it leaves a lot faster. If you're willing to march right up to yourself and feel what's going on inside, what you find on the other side is a reward. Fire races through the muscle. Skin tightens, veins pulsate. You are full and engorged, with a post-orgasmic sort of high. You get braver, lay on another paper-thin coat of strength and grant yourself the opportunity to conquer discomfort and fear. You become more resilient inside. Turning discomfort into pleasure is an alchemical process, which can teach you to master emotional discomforts—and walk a cleaner path through life without laying your feelings over those who find themselves in your way.

Breathing

When syncing the breath with each repetition, exhale as the weight lifts, inhale as it lowers. The exhalation increases intra-abdominal pressure and acts as an internal brace for the whole body. An easy way to remember is *ex*-hale with *ex*-ertion.

I'm not sure why, but most people do this backwards. If it's too hard to sync the exhalations with each lift, just breathe naturally. It's tempting to hold the breath when training gets hard—and an occasional held breath is okay (and natural) during the hardest part of a lift. But holding it too long could cause a dangerous condition called a Valsalva maneuver, which, among other things, reduces blood flow to the heart, cuts down oxygen to the brain and can make you dizzy or even pass out!

Breathing offers a way to refuel. Think of blowing the weight up on a pocket of air. Or pause in a long breath between reps to gather strength and complete the set.

Stretch Between Sets

Resting between sets lets you recover, regroup, frame each exercise with thought, begin again. Rest time should last about as long as it takes to do an exercise. Yet instead of talking or spacing out during rests, use ballet or yoga-inspired stretches to take muscles from contraction into an elongated state of surrender. This adds yin to yang, complements the contraction and minimizes the soreness that occurs one or two days after training.

I like gravity-assisted stretches—hanging off a Smith Machine bar, holding on to a fixed pole and stretching away from it or draping my spine over a Physioball (a giant rubber ball). Regardless of where, when or how you stretch, you get the most benefit when muscles are already warm and pliant. Muscles are like taffy. Pulling a piece of cold taffy makes it snap in two, but hot taffy keeps on stretching.

I also head to the pool at least once a week for a long bout of yoga-type stretches. Since body weight is so greatly diminished in water, it's much easier to "float" the limbs into positions that would be hard to do on land. Wearing buoyant ankle cuffs gives extra buoyancy. (See "More Tools and Toys for Transformation" for more information.)

Periodization

Some people like to train for weeks at a time in a particular rep range—a technique called "periodization" borrowed from pro athletes. A typical cycle would use up to 6 weeks for low reps, followed by 6 for moderate reps, then 6 more for high reps. The idea once again is to work different types of muscle fibers and prepare for a specific event. This may make sense for an athlete in training. But for the woman who is simply "training for life," 6 weeks of one style of training could get tiresome and even lead to overuse injuries—particularly if she's not strong enough to go through the power phase.

It also doesn't allow for varying moods, energy levels and the hormonal changes that sometimes lead you on roller-coaster rides through monthly cycles. It may work best simply to vary the reps and weight according to how you feel on a given day—or even within one workout.

The Splits

Muscles grow in recovery—not during workouts. "Hitting 'em hard" again the next day interferes with recovery and thus can hinder progress. However, light, gentle motions the next day for those same body parts can increase blood flow, warming and soothing stiff muscles. But it's wise to wait at least 48 hours before doing an intense workout for the same muscles.

There's no end to the variations you can use to split up your body parts and no need to stick with one "split." When you start to feel like a hamster on a wheel, stuck in a routine, it's time to change things around. There are many standard "splits," but the best split is the one you create yourself.

THE BASIC BEGINNER, WHOLE BODY WORKOUT

Mon, Wed, Sat—

or Tues, Thurs, Sat—whole body

Alternate exercises and rep ranges with at least every other workout.

Aerobics 3 to 5 days a week.

The much-praised "full body workout" is valuable for getting started, coming back after a layoff and maintenance, but isn't the most effective way to improve. Its value is more psychological than physical. You get the assurance that in the course of an hour, every muscle group was addressed—and you may have thrown in your aerobics, too—doing every nasty deed all at once. This appeals to our time-crunched society but isn't the true road to muscle mastery. Here, it is much more valuable to "divide and conquer."

A STANDARD ADVANCED BEGINNER SPLIT

Mon, Thurs—upper body and abs

Tues, Fri—lower body

Try heavier weights, fewer reps at the beginning of the week (when energy is greater)—and lighter weights, more reps at the end.

Aerobics 3 to 5 days a week.

THE BASIC THREE-DAY SPLIT

Mon—chest, shoulders, triceps and abs

Tues—legs and calves

Wed—back, biceps and abs

Thurs—rest

Fri—begin again . . . but with a slightly different approach, different
angles, exercises, reps

Aerobics 3 to 5 days a week.

(Personally, I find this routine gets old very fast.)

A FOUR-DAY SPLIT

Mon—back, rear delts and abs

Tues—legs

Wed—chest and shoulders

Thurs—biceps, triceps and abs

Fri—rest

Sat—begin again

Aerobics 3 to 5 days a week.

A QUIRKY FIVE-DAY SPLIT (MY SPLIT)

Mon—back, rear delts and abs

Tues—quads, inner and outer thigh

Wed—chest, shoulders and abs

Thurs—rest

Friday—hamstrings, gluteus, calves

Saturday—biceps, triceps and abs

Sunday—rest

Aerobics 3 to 5 days a week.

Some people might not believe that advances can be made working
each major muscle group only once a week. However, I've made more
gains this way than when I trained each part twice a week. My training is
more focused now, and this also leaves plenty of time for recovery (I'm

also a hard gainer—with long limbs. If I overdo my training, I defeat my own goals.) Technically, however, many muscle groups actually get worked twice—though not directly. For instance, triceps assist in chest workouts, biceps in back workouts, and quads and gluteus get worked in many of the leg exercises.

I also supplement my training with other types of movement. In addition to traditional aerobics (on a bike, stairs, running, fast walking, etc.), I also do water exercise (deep and shallow running, swimming, and a series of spiraling motions I call water tai chi), which rejuvenates my muscles, mind and spirit.

OPPOSING MUSCLE GROUPS

Mon—upper back, chest and shoulders

Tues—gluteus, outer and inner thigh, lower back and abs

Wed—biceps, triceps, forearms

Thurs—quads, hamstrings, calves

Friday—rest

Saturday—rest or begin again

Aerobics 3 to 5 days a week.

AN "ON THE RUN" SPLIT (CATCH IT WHEN YOU CAN)

Mon am—20 minutes back, 10 min. abs

Mon pm—30 min. brisk walk

Tues am—30–40 min. legs

Tues pm—10 min. stretch and abs

Wed am—30 min. chest and shoulders

30 min. aerobics

Thurs—water aerobics and stretch

Friday—30 min. biceps and triceps

Saturday—45 min. bike ride

Sunday—hike, play, whatever

Although this last one looks like a lot of exercise, it isn't really. It's easier to do a little bit every day, or even twice a day, than to save it up for a few days a week. After all, you eat every day, breathe, walk, think—why not exercise? Taking a day off every once in a while is important when you're tired. But taking off too many days in a row (unless you're sick or recovering) takes its toll—especially as you get older. It's that much harder to crank it up all over again.

Also, after a two- to three-week layoff from weight training, muscles lose about 10% to 15% of their strength. However, once you build strength and lose it, it takes less time to get it back. So when you have to stop for a while, at least you know you can pick it up again faster. This truism is known as "muscle memory," and many trainees have experienced this in action. Still, it doesn't help to wait too long.

Aerobics and Training

Training takes a fresh state of mind and a full store of energy. Personally, I can't do aerobics first and then have enough energy left to sustain a weight workout. I need my mind and body fresh. Yet some people say they need the rush and heat of aerobics to warm them up for training.

It makes sense to me to use up the carbohydrates stored from breakfast or last night's dinner for weight workouts, since that's the main fuel used in weight training. Presumably, once those carbohydrates (or glycogen) are depleted, you can more rapidly dip into the "fat stores" and use *that* to fuel the aerobics. Otherwise you spend 20 minutes of aerobic time just to use up glycogen before getting to the fat.

Plus, after the focus of training, it's a relief to "space out" on a stationary bike or stair machine and read. It doesn't much matter if the muscles are fatigued or if the brain is fully engaged to do this. But you have to keep in mind your main objective. If you want strength, definition, optimal muscle function and to lose body fat, then resistance training would be the first priority. If you're in training for an endurance event, then the main focus would be on aerobics, with weights as a supplement.

So the question is, when to fit the aerobic portion in? Either immediately after training (or before, if you must), later on that day or on different days. You need a minimum of three aerobic workouts per week, 20 to 40 minutes each, to maintain cardiovascular conditioning and promote more fat loss.

Go Out and Play

If all this sounds like no fun, there are alternatives for the "aerobically unchallenged." To levitate out of the mundane 20- to 40-minute prescription of sweat and punishment on a piece of machinery, give yourself a dose of play. There's no shortage of options if you're just willing to break out of habit.

Some aerobic alternatives:

- Hikes or vigorous walks—to air out your brain, look around, appreciate the scenery, let inspiration come. To up the intensity, hike hills or walk briskly with big arm motions.

- Deep water exercise—or "aqua jogging" wearing a flotation belt, optional footgear and possibly a waterproof pouch for a Walkman—to boogie in the deep! (For more information see "More Tools and Toys for Transformation.") This 3-D resistance lets you float and fly as in a dream, while pushing and pulling the viscous density of the water, thus getting three workouts in one— aerobics, moderate muscle conditioning and stretching, with zero impact on the joints. Quite a workout, and a bit like dancing in air!

- Rock or wall climbing—a good sport for recovering acrophobics. This sport literally takes you out on the edge, while securely roping you in at the same time. An incredible workout for upper body, legs and mind, and a test of courage.

- In-line skating. A good quad workout, test of balance and agility—a natural for speed demons and the fearless among us. Pad up.

- Swimming variations: Vary lengths of freestyle, with backstroke, breaststroke, upper body only (using a pull buoy) and legs only (using kickboards). Increase upper body strength by adding webbed gloves; increase speed by wearing short flippers.

- Running variations: Jog, skip, hop, chassé, slide side to side as if on skates, go backwards, sideways, walk, run full-out to that telephone pole, walk again, lift knees in a high march, kick heels to butt, land in the center of each sidewalk square, boogie to a favorite song— and never mind what the neighbors say.

- Play with some kids in a playground—swing, hang, climb, slide, jump rope, hopscotch.

- Take an African or Brazilian dance class. "Get down" into the Earth-Mama pelvis, make full contact with the floor in bare feet, let the rhythm move through the body and dance full-out to the beat.

Plateaus and Valleys

When training to improve, you should see results every three months. However, it's not possible to improve all the time. Sometimes you've got to "catch up with yourself," process the information, go into maintenance mode or even backslide a while. In fact, it's important to take mental breathers like this, pulling back into a kind of "active rest." But when it's time to rev it up again, shake up a dull routine or push to the next level, you don't have to do everything at once. Try experimenting with various aspects of training—making one change at a time. Plug each one in separately, in a modular fashion to see what actually works:

To shake up a weight routine, try:

- changing splits

- adding or *subtracting* an extra day (to avoid overdoing it)

- using heavier weights

- doing more repetitions with lighter weights or

- taking shorter rests between sets.

To shake up an aerobic routine, try:

- adding 1 or 2 more days of aerobics per week

- adding an extra 10 minutes to 1 or 2 aerobic workouts per week—to increase duration

- intervals, to push up the intensity and increase aerobic capacity (just be careful not to get completely out of breath). Try mixing periods of various intensities (such as "moderate, somewhat hard and hard") for 30 seconds to 3 minutes each.

- a different style of workout or

- something that really makes you *sweat.*

To shake up eating habits, try:

- smaller meals, more often throughout the day to keep your metabolism "stoked"

- eating more calories but less fat

- cutting out addictions to junk—replacing them with healthy substitutes or, at least, healthier junk.

What You Can Expect on This Journey: Romance and Commitment

At first when you start training, it's like dating. It's easy to feel flush with excitement and possibilities—combined with twinges of awkwardness and virgin soreness. You might not see results right away but underneath the surface, a new awareness takes hold, a new hardness appears under your skin. Old aches disappear. New ones take their place. After a few weeks or months, little mounds of muscle start to appear. Fat begins to fade away. And if you're already lean, lines of definition begin to etch themselves across your skin. Things start to change.

In a matter of weeks or months, your strength doubles and triples, your confidence soars. You feel proud, puffed up with potential. You may feel like a convert and try to convince your friends—yet find that few share your enthusiasm. So, you sail off on your own journey, leaving some friends behind, finding new ones and gliding along on a feeling of adventure.

You may hire trainers, subscribe to muscle magazines, buy lifting belts, gloves and all sorts of supplements without knowing what they do (if anything). You may spy on others who seem to know what they're doing, and try out their exercises. You may even radically change your diet—eating oatmeal and egg whites for breakfast, lots of white tuna and chicken breast without skin—and find yourself speaking less in terms of "pizza" and "ice cream" and more in terms of "carbs," "proteins" and grams of fat. After brushing your teeth in the morning, you might even pose and flex in the bathroom mirror—and like what you see.

Months go by. The relationship begins to run into a little trouble—an ache grows here, an injury there. You may have spent a big chunk of salary on supplements—but no new changes have appeared. The gains that were hot and fast may now slow down—even reverse! The routine feels boring, and you find yourself stretched out on a vast desert where nothing seems to be happening at all. You're parched, dry, cranky, and those last five pounds won't budge.

At this point, you might move on. The average gym membership lasts about three to four months—about the time it takes for the romance to fade. The obvious justification is that training doesn't suit you. It's dull, repetitive and too far from home. But it isn't training, per se, that doesn't suit. The hard part about training is the commitment—not to weight lifting but to anything. For many, this is *the* glitch, the same place where you blow it every time, fracture your bonds, pull up roots and head on out, looking for "it," when "it" may be under your nose the whole time. At some point, you realize that you must wake up every day with training somewhere on the horizon—even if it's a day off. For some, this reality is too much to bear. It's no longer new, enticing. This is when things truly get scary because, just as in a relationship that loses its luster, you begin to feel stuck in it forever. Your eyes start to wander. Can you make it over the hump?

Some may stay in it grudgingly just for the dangling carrot of *results* (thinking, "Why else would I put myself through this self-inflicted torture?"). Many others may wonder, "Where's this 'pump' I've heard about? And where are my muscles?'' Some people take steroids not just for the muscle growth, but for the constant rush of "go get 'em" motivation.

Sometimes hanging around a gym can be discouraging, too, especially if you absorb all the unsolicited advice. When someone recommends this or that supplement or training technique, you may run around like a rat in a maze, chasing some elusive goal that may not have been your intention in the first place. And if someone happens to say you haven't got "the genetics" for what you're trying to achieve—your poor striving heart may reel in despair and give it all up, thinking, "If the genetic deck is stacked against me, why bother?" Genetics do determine body "structure." But every single body out there, as well as every mind, can be improved with weight training. Believing in the fairy tale that there are certain "genetically gifted" superior beings (which, of course, you aren't one of) is the road to misery. Even if it's true (and I think this is highly debatable, since athletes aren't born but made), it's best to either ignore it altogether, or imagine yourself as part of that elite group.

There are other valleys of despair in the iron game, too. It gets lonely. No one can lift that weight for you, and no one feels your pain. It doesn't help if your friends and family think you've gone off your rocker for pumping iron, or your lover starts to feel jealous of barbells. It's a challenge to stay true to your self-commitment, without alienating others.

It's also wise to avoid the trap of obsession. Chances are, anyone who is smitten with training will confront this. The art of muscle sculpting even just for health reasons tends to draw high-achieving individuals— often ones with perfectionist tendencies. When such perfection doesn't happen (and it never does to your standards—plus it's slow, slow, slow), the tendency is either to drive even harder—or else pull the plug, quit, overeat and seek balance by running the other way. This same pattern often plays itself out in relationships, too, when they turn the dangerous corner from romance to commitment. The temptation is either to force it to work or abandon ship, reclaim your freedom, even jump on another shining opportunity—another person, another sport, another promise, thinking maybe *they've* got what you need. In both a training program and a relationship, this is the critical stage. You can continue to repeat this on-and-off cycle, or you can ride out the discomfort and this time, perhaps, experience breakthrough.

Like mature love, training works its most profound magic not in a hot, quick romance, but in a long-term relationship—and like marriage, it needs to be invented over and over to keep itself evolving and alive. From time to time, you need to pull back and reassess, look at your workouts as you might well look at your spouse—not as a predictable dullard farting around the house—but as a miracle, a mystery you may never fully explore, not to be dreaded but embraced. It's easy to think you have it all figured out. But there's always something new to discover. Sometimes all it takes is a fresh eye, a vivid imagination and a renewed sense of appreciation to build the magic again. If you imbue the experience with special powers, chances are better they'll show up. If not, chances are slim indeed.

For those who ride out these rocky phases, backslide, fall off and get back on the horse when times are tough, the rewards are sweet. What may have started as a sexy, fiery, "she's gotta have it" passion in the muscles can mature into the sheer pleasure of motion and the joy of one's own company. The passion is still there—in fact it grows, but it takes a back seat. It's no longer the motivator, the glue that holds you together or gives you a rush or a high. The real pleasure comes from the humble, daily act of building and creating the experience for yourself anew—and the riches rise off the *consistent* application of imagination and love. After a while, it's not just the body that gets built, but concentration, dedication, the profound pleasure of simple actions, repeated over and over as if in prayer. This time alone inside one's experience can be the high point of the day, a sanctuary from outside madness. Sometimes the hard part, in fact, becomes going back *into* the world.

When I hit rough spots in my training, I try to forget what I think I know and start fresh, questioning everything. Actually, I try to do this every day! Instead of the same old, same old, I may do the exercises in reverse order, work with equipment I seldom use or find a new running trail, pop a different cassette in my Walkman, try workouts at a completely different time of day, breaking the routine.

I forget about "getting a workout" and instead just play. This takes the pressure off "building muscle," "burning calories" or achieving anything "important" and frees my imagination. It lets me wander like a wide-eyed tourist in new territory—rather than a jaded old-timer down the same old block. By releasing my obsession about "having to train" (which can become a burden), I free my otherwise rigid, over-achieving personality. The pressure drops immediately. I have a much better time and usually end up getting a much better workout.

Other times, when I don't feel "fully present," I put me aside completely and instead, literally "zip myself" into the skin of my idealized self, a character from my imagination. She's taller, stronger, more thoughtful and better-looking than I am. She doesn't complain and works in silence, oblivious to what others think. She doesn't care how her hair looks (which, regardless, is always great) or if her stomach sticks out (which, of course, it never does!). She's always grounded, polite and naturally poised, and she takes each set right up to the wall and beyond—turning pain into pleasure, making games out of each motion. She's strong as a Viking, intelligent, intense. She channels her energy wisely, never wasting even so much as a word. Ripples of muscle brush across her skin as she moves. She seems to dwell inside a golden glow—and others around her respect this boundary, don't intrude.

With her in charge, all I have to do is take orders. She's the one who chooses the exercises and coaches me with just the right words. She lends me her strength, concentration and grace—every little detail, right down to how she holds her head and breathes. If it weren't for her, I'd probably spend too much time blabbing between sets and gazing around the room. She keeps me in line and supports me in becoming like her. She's patient with my shortcomings and she's gracious, too, letting me borrow her strong points while I reap all the rewards.

Self-Assessment:
The Body Puzzle

Evaluations

Before embarking, find out if you're a "high risk" candidate for training. A good personal trainer, for instance, would ask you these questions:

- Is your blood pressure greater than or equal to 160/90? _____

- Is your total cholesterol greater or equal to 240? _____

- Do you smoke? _____

- Do you have diabetes? _____

- Do you have a family history of heart disease? _____

- Cancer? _____

- Do you live a sedentary lifestyle? _____

- Are you over 50? (for females—for men it's over 40) _____

- Are you pregnant? _____

- Are you on medications? _____

- Is your body fat over 30 percent? _____

- Do you have a known disease? _____

- Do you have any old or recent injuries? _____

If you answered yes to two or more of the above questions, the American College of Sports Medicine recommends that you get your doctor's clearance before starting.

You'll also need to evaluate your schedule to see how many days a week you can realistically train—and thus divide up your workouts accordingly. (See "Sample Workouts," page 202.)

Find out your measurements and percentage of body fat. This gives you a more accurate picture of your body composition than just weighing in. (Once you start putting on muscle, body weight can often *increase*, since muscle weighs more than fat—and this can mislead you into thinking you're not making progress when you are.) Start with these measurements, which you can update every 6 weeks to 3 months to chart progress. Example:

date: _____

% body fat _____

body weight _____

measurements:

chest (pectoral, just above breasts) _____

waist _____

hips (at hip bone) _____

buttocks (the biggest part! keep feet together) _____

thigh (uppermost section) _____

calves _____

biceps (around the most bulbous part) _____

(Dropping body fat levels by 1% to 3% every six weeks, during a "losing phase," is a nice comfortable pace. Allow yourself 6 weeks to 3 months to feel and see if your workouts are working.)

Next, try to evaluate your postural weaknesses and imbalances in a detached, preferably nonjudgmental way. If you can't do this evaluation yourself, have someone snap a photo of you from front, back and sides—or have *them* do the assessment. Draw two bodies, one straight-on and one in profile. Mark each area of imbalance with an X and R or L for right or left.

Although all of the above details can touch at the heart of paranoia and make the head reel with self-judgment, the facts give you a place to begin. It takes a certain type of courage to embrace the less glamorous side of reality—but all improvements spring from there.

Posture

- Do you tilt your head to one side? _____
  (Do you cradle a phone on your neck? _____)

- Is one shoulder higher than the other? _____
  (Do you always carry a bag on the same side? _____)

- Do you tend to slump forward? _____
  (Do you sit at a desk all day? _____)

- Does your chest sink in? _____

- Do you strain your neck forward when you read or write? _____

- Do you have a pronounced arch in your lower back (lordosis)? _____

- Do you have scoliosis? _____

- Do you know which sides of the spine are overstretched or contracted, due to the scoliosis? _____

- Is one leg longer than the other? _____ Which one? _____

- Do you lean into one hip? _____

- Do your knees bow out or knock together? _____

- Do you lock your knees when standing? _____

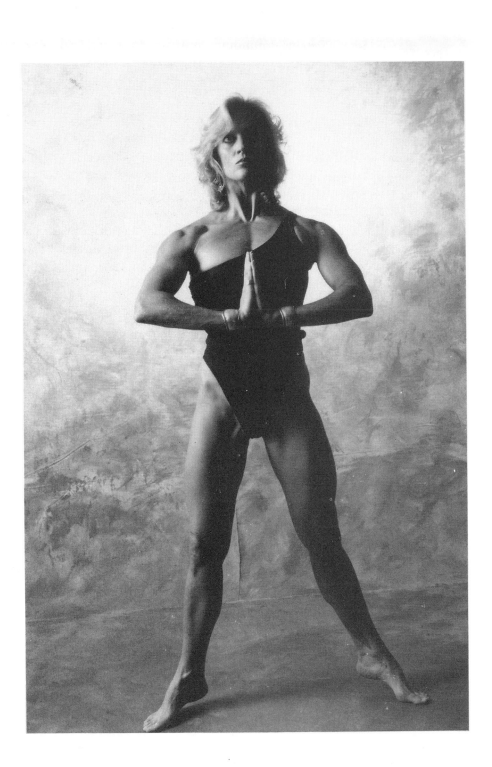

- Do you wear high heels much of the time? _____
  (If so, your Achilles tendons could become tight and "shortened.")

- Do your feet roll in or out? _____
  (Check the wear on the soles of your shoes to see.)

Some of these things can be fixed with a shift in posture or changing habits. Fixing others requires strengthening weak muscles and lengthening or stretching tight ones.

Some Postural Fixes

- Tilt head to one side
  Stretch neck muscles on the "shorter side" and try to carry head straight

- Shoulders slump forward
  Strengthen the "rear" part of shoulder and upper back

- Arched lower back (lordosis) or weakness in lower back and the abdominals
  Strengthen abdominals
  Stretch (and strengthen) lower back muscles
  Strengthen (and stretch) weak hamstrings
  "Soften" locked knees
  Lengthen and increase mobility of hip flexors with hip flexor stretches
  Incorporate balance exercises (such as standing on one leg) to improve torso stabilizing muscles, posture and alignment

- Flat lower back with shoulders rounded forward (kyphosis)
  Strengthen rear shoulder and upper back muscles to correct slumping
  Strengthen chest to open posture
  Stretch (and strengthen) tight hamstrings
  Strengthen hip flexors while maintaining flexibility in that muscle

- Feet rolling in or out
  Possible candidate for orthotics (corrective inserts for shoes), particularly if you run or do any type of impact exercise, which would

exacerbate the problem. Try focusing on centering your weight through the whole foot.

- For tight Achilles tendons

  Try walking barefoot in sand. Or stretch your Achilles tendons by standing on stairs, lowering one heel and slightly bending the knee on that leg at the same time.

- To break the habit of always carrying a bag on one side

  Switch sides or carry a backpack

- To minimize neck pain

  Make sure you don't cradle the phone in your neck. Get a headset or shoulder brace. Try a speaker phone.

- If you slump at a desk all day

  Treat yourself to an ergonomic chair with good lower back support

- Scoliosis

  People often ask me if I encountered any great pain or difficulty with my scoliosis or had to develop a "special workout." I improved my scoliosis simply by strengthening my back muscles. I didn't do any "special" scoliosis workouts. I simply started with pull downs and seated rows, concentrating on pulling with equal force on both sides, to "educate" my back muscles how to pull in a balanced way, without favoring the stronger side. Later I added extra reps on my weaker sides (my right upper back and left lower back) with exercises such as one-arm rows and rear delt exercises with dumbbells. I also made sure to stretch the "bunched up" stronger sides.

  I also spent a lot of time hanging upside down—and still do. The first time I did this I had someone run a hand down my spine and discovered that by reversing the direction of gravity's effect on my body, I almost straightened out my spine! I figured that if it could be straight when upside down, it could be straight when right side up, too. So I set out to "program" my spine to remember what straight felt like (a slight shift to the right in my rib cage, a slight bend in the left knee). I'm now a believer in the benefits of "inversion" and make sure to practice this daily. (For a list of inversion devices, see "Tools and Toys.") However, inversion isn't for everybody. Going too quickly upside down can be dangerous (and scary) if you're not used to it. Check with a chiropractor to see if it's right for you.

I've since worked with several people with varying degrees of curvature. Each has to make individual adjustments in posture to find what feels "straight." However, the two arm, then one arm method described above, plus stretching, seems to work for all.

Muscle Checklist

Next, try to flex each muscle (hardening and softening). Do this as if you were showing off your biceps. Bend or straighten appropriate limbs to contract the muscles. The ones that fail to take your orders are the ones that probably need your most attention.

- What muscles fail to harden at your command?

shoulders	____	biceps	____	quads	____
chest	____	triceps	____	hamstrings	____
back (lats)	____	abdominals	____	inner thigh	____
lower back	____	buttocks	____	calves	____

- Do you have any old or current injuries that require nurturing and respect? Where?

  _____ _____ _____

  _____ _____ _____

- What sorts of physical activities do you do now? (Either athletic or not)

  _____ _____ _____

  _____ _____ _____

- What body parts or muscles do those activities use most?

  _____ _____ _____

  _____ _____ _____

- What parts, therefore, do you use least? What needs more attention?

  _____ _____ _____

  _____ _____ _____

Use your weak and neglected areas as focal points for training. Don't simply start by favoring what you already do well. Fill in the missing pieces of your puzzle—and a weak muscle can soon become a strong point.

- For instance, if you do a lot of step classes or the stair machine, you get lots of hip flexor, buttocks and quadriceps work, but very little hamstring and upper body work.

  To create balance, strengthen hamstrings and upper body, lengthen and stretch tight hip flexors.

- If you play tennis, you're probably stronger on one side.

  Work on bringing up your weaker side. Also, you may need more quadriceps work to increase "crouch power," more pain-free shoulder rotation to improve your serve (stretch and strengthen external rotators) and more aerobics to improve endurance, since tennis is often a stop-and-go (anaerobic) sport, which, therefore, doesn't contribute much to metabolizing fat for fuel or improving cardiovascular endurance.

- If you're a swimmer, with plenty of upper body strength, you probably need more leg exercises for strength and aesthetics, since flutter kicks don't work legs through a large range of motion (and therefore don't sculpt the gluteus). Also, since swimming is non-weight bearing, it doesn't harden the bones the way weight training can.

  Add full range-of-motion leg exercises, in the water and out, and add weight training in general as a long-term investment for your bones. Concentrating on back and chest work will improve your strokes. Just be sure not to overtrain shoulders with heavy weight, as that could cause injury and hamper your swimming altogether.

- If you're a runner/walker, chances are good you only work the lower half of your body.

  Add upper body strengthening to address neglected muscles. You might even need supplemental leg training to improve leg strength and endurance—especially hamstring and quads for hip and knee stability. To sculpt buttocks, add exercises for that area and sprint up hills to improve both your shape and aerobic capacity. If you suffer from overuse injuries from running, run in both deep and shallow water. If it's a serious injury, start in deep and work into progressively shallower water, where you weigh more, so you gradually overload muscles and joints.

Part Three
The Exercises

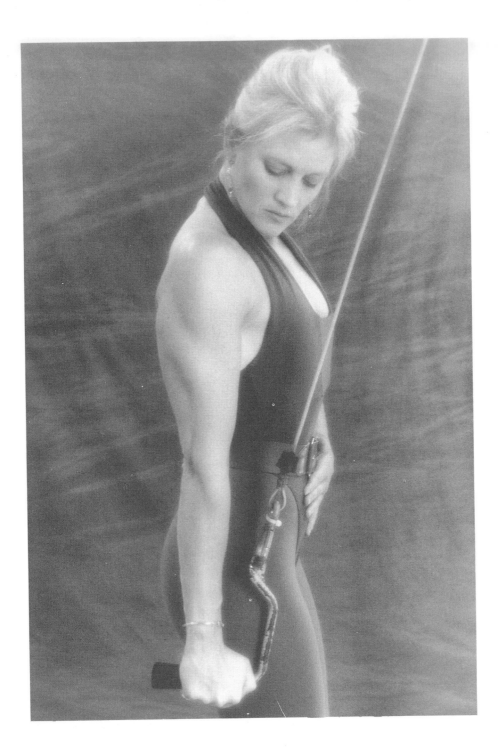

The Shifting Truth

OUR KNOWLEDGE of exercise is perpetually unfolding. Every month in almost every health and fitness publication, new research and discoveries confirm or contradict old beliefs. In weight training, in particular, there's a great deal of emerging research, an abundance of controversy and no shortage of "gray areas." Some of the "truths" are hard to pin down, since what's true for me may not be true for you. Even many "experts" often can't agree on how to do exercises, which ones are safe, what muscles get worked, how many sets or reps to do and how often to train.

There's a good deal of inexactness to this artful science and much folklore and tradition as well. The motto in many gyms is "Lift heavy, train hard, eat carbs for energy and protein for muscle growth and you will succeed," which to a certain extent is true. But I know several "old-timers" who have trained this way for decades, have good muscles to show for it, but never give their bodies a chance to recoup with lighter weight or a different training style—and limp around with bad knees, hips, backs and shoulders.

Intelligent weight training should be an ongoing experiment—questioning both the "old school" basic training methods and the latest research. Neither holds the gospel truth that works for each of you.

Therefore, I present my own methods, culled from eight years of working with hundreds of people, years of study, workshops, certifications, reading, reviewing scientific data, conducting experiments on myself to test the effectiveness of various exercises, constant practice, deductive reasoning and common sense. I'm aware that each person is unique and that all exercises can't work for all people. I'm also aware that time and new information may outdate some of what is here. However, I'm counting on the facts that gravity will always make things fall down and bodies will continue to be put together the same way.

I encourage you to keep asking questions, dig for the truth that is your own and make any adjustments you need so these exercises work for you.

How to Choose Exercises from This Book

All exercises marked "Basic Exercise" are good for both beginners and seasoned trainers. Add the intermediate and advanced exercises only after you've developed good core strength, have an understanding of form, and feel confident with your ability.

Most of the equipment shown here is standard and found in most gyms. If you work out at home and don't have access to machines, stick with the free weight exercises (i.e., barbells and dumbbells) and do the standing leg work and exercises that don't require large pieces of equipment. You may also want to invest in a pair of 1 to 5 pound or adjustable ankle weights for the hamstring, buttocks, inner and outer thigh exercises that mention ankle weights. For cable exercises, you can use elastic resistance bands such as Dyna-bands, surgical tubing, or a "Lifeline Gym" (a tubing device with handles and other accessories, available in sporting goods stores). However, to mimic the cable movements, you will have to anchor one end of the elastic underfoot, hold it overhead or tie it to a pole, so you have a fixed point and pull against it. Remember to pull the band in one direction only for maximum resistance. (You can also order my Dyna-Gym video which shows an all-over band workout.)

The exercise-anatomy chart shows you which muscles you'll be working on.

Exercise Symbol Key

Move in this direction

Press down here

Clock face to guide movement

Lift up here

90 degree angle of joint

Main moving joint

Soft, slightly bent joint

Dead zone

End movement here

Maintain natural curve of spine

Line up joints this way

Keep back parallel to floor

EXERCISE-ANATOMY CHART

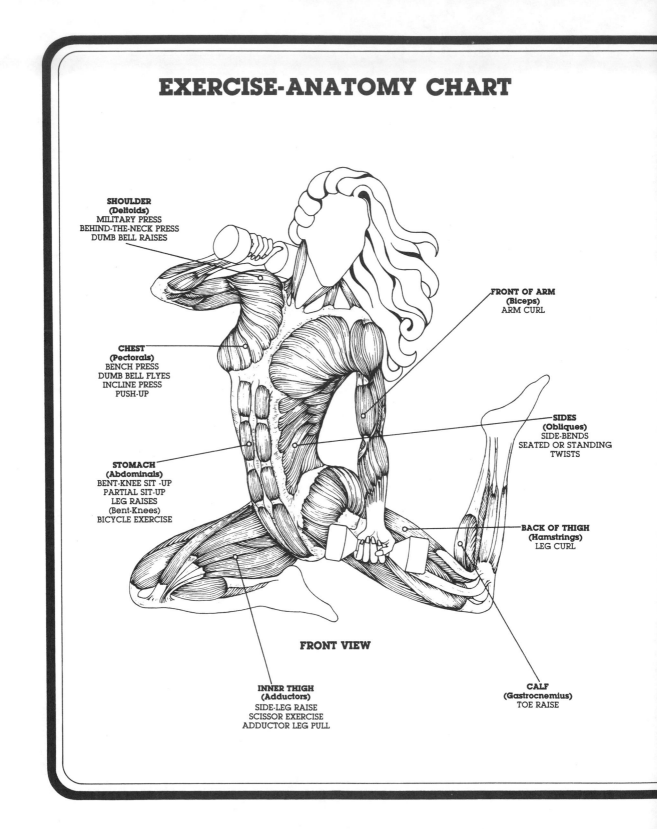

SHOULDER
(Deltoids)
MILITARY PRESS
BEHIND-THE-NECK PRESS
DUMB BELL RAISES

FRONT OF ARM
(Biceps)
ARM CURL

CHEST
(Pectorals)
BENCH PRESS
DUMB BELL FLYES
INCLINE PRESS
PUSH-UP

SIDES
(Obliques)
SIDE-BENDS
SEATED OR STANDING
TWISTS

STOMACH
(Abdominals)
BENT-KNEE SIT -UP
PARTIAL SIT-UP
LEG RAISES
(Bent-Knees)
BICYCLE EXERCISE

BACK OF THIGH
(Hamstrings)
LEG CURL

FRONT VIEW

INNER THIGH
(Adductors)
SIDE-LEG RAISE
SCISSOR EXERCISE
ADDUCTOR LEG PULL

CALF
(Gastrocnemius)
TOE RAISE

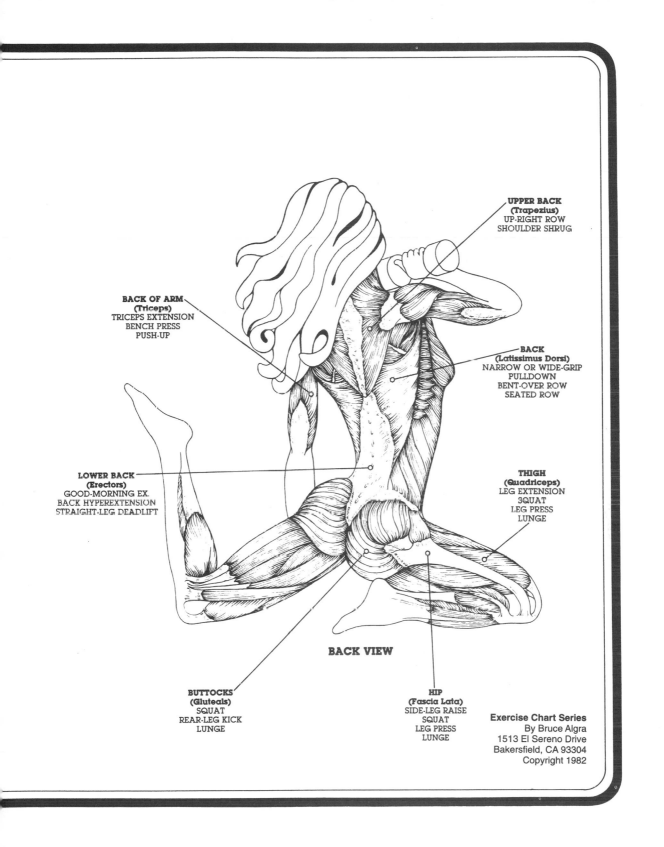

UPPER BACK
(Trapezius)
UP-RIGHT ROW
SHOULDER SHRUG

BACK OF ARM
(Triceps)
TRICEPS EXTENSION
BENCH PRESS
PUSH-UP

BACK
(Latissimus Dorsi)
NARROW OR WIDE-GRIP
PULLDOWN
BENT-OVER ROW
SEATED ROW

LOWER BACK
(Erectors)
GOOD-MORNING EX.
BACK HYPEREXTENSION
STRAIGHT-LEG DEADLIFT

THIGH
(Quadriceps)
LEG EXTENSION
SQUAT
LEG PRESS
LUNGE

BACK VIEW

BUTTOCKS
(Gluteals)
SQUAT
REAR-LEG KICK
LUNGE

HIP
(Fascia Lata)
SIDE-LEG RAISE
SQUAT
LEG PRESS
LUNGE

Exercise Chart Series
By Bruce Algra
1513 El Sereno Drive
Bakersfield, CA 93304
Copyright 1982

Leg Exercises

Exercise 1   Leg Press

BASIC EXERCISE   This is a good strengthening and re-shaping exercise for people who don't like regular free bar squats with weight compressing the spine.

Movement   Adjust the back rest of the machine if you can to approximately 45 degrees (lower doesn't give your back adequate support, higher "squashes" your internal organs and shortens your motion). Place your feet high on the plate, with your toes over the edge, so that when your knees lower, they don't exceed a 90-degree angle and your heels stay on the plate. Lower the plate *slowly*, holding on to the handles. As you straighten your legs, press with your *heels* and keep your knees "soft" to keep the workload in your muscles, not the joints.

Drawing with the weight   Keep watch over your thighs—they should stay parallel to each other throughout. Don't knock or bow your knees. Also, if you have a side mirror, watch that your knees make clean right angles. Slightly less is okay for beginners, slightly more is fine for intermediates, as long as your feet are high on the plate and your motion is controlled.

Safety tips   Keep your lower back in neutral—not arching or pelvic-tilting into pad. Aim for a full range of motion here but beware of "dropping" the weight into your knees and banging your thighs into your chest. Always use a weight you can handle so you can achieve full range of motion. There's no need to use heavy weight and lower only halfway down. It mostly benefits the ego—and uses some quadriceps—but does nothing for the buttocks!

Targeted muscles   Quadriceps, inner thigh and buttocks. (Note: If you move your feet lower down on the plate, hamstrings contribute a little more but still not much—and it's problematic for knees.) Putting your feet higher on the plate activates more gluteus, as does using a slightly deeper range of motion.

Main moving joints   Knee and hip.

Function   Basic leg strength for walking, climbing, running, bounding.

Aesthetics   Adds a slight, shapely sweep to the thighs (doesn't make them huge, however!). Also adds tone to the inner thigh and helps raise and round the buttocks.

Tricks of the trade   Lower the plate very slowly—to the count of 10. Then press up in 1 or 2—but remember not to "lock out" the knees. This "works the negative" and takes a high level of control—good for penetrating deep into more muscle fibers.

Leg Exercises

REMINDERS:

1. Avoid "dropping" weight into knees
2. Keep legs parallel
3. Aim for 90-degree knee angle
4. Press with heels
5. Don't "lock out" knees

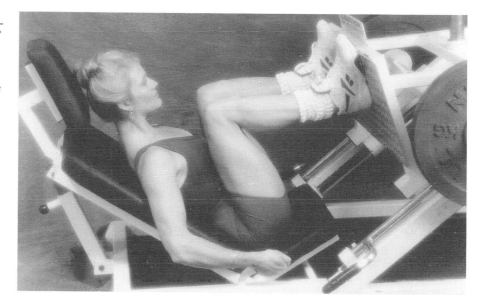

No cheating Don't push your knees with your hands, until absolutely necessary. That's your ace in the hole.

Visualization Imagine you have a 6″ brace between your knees to keep them in constant relation to each other at all times. Let your legs draw two parallel lines.

Variation One leg at a time. Often you'll need less than half of what you'd use with both legs. (Balance on two limbs gives you the advantage of leverage.) Or try this with a wide leg position, feet slightly turned out (as in a ballet 2nd position), making sure your knees don't press out over your ankles.

Leg Exercises

Exercise 2   Sit-Back Squats

BASIC EXERCISE, modified to make it easier on the back

Unlike free bar squats, which put forward force into the lower back and knees, here the force travels back into the hips and buttocks—where it's needed, without compromising vulnerable areas.

Movement

Grab onto a fixed pole (or something that won't move). Bring your feet 1 to 3 inches from the pole, so that when you *sit back into your hips* your back is vertical (as if you were sitting in a straight-back Victorian chair). Extend your arms. If your feet are too far from the pole, you'll lean forward. You should feel that if someone took the pole away, you'd fall backward. Your lower thighs should be parallel to the floor, or just slightly lower than that. (This won't bother your knees, since the force is traveling backwards.) As you lift, press your weight into your *heels*. LIFT ONLY HALFWAY UP to keep the workload in the buttocks.

Drawing with the weight

The weight you're lifting is your torso. Keep it in a solid vertical. At the bottom of the motion, your knees, hips and back all form 90-degree angles.

Safety tips

Make sure your back stays upright—no rounding. Lower with control, so you don't "drop" into your hips. Also avoid coming up all the way, locking your knees.

Targeted muscles

Buttocks, quads and inner thighs.

Main moving joints

Hips and knees.

Function

Basic leg strength for climbing, walking, running and many sports.

Aesthetics

Adds rounded firmness to buttocks and inner thigh, also shape to frontal thigh.

Tricks of the trade

Lift your toes to make sure you're pressing into your heels. Once your shin muscles fatigue, then rest the toes and use the mind.

No cheating

Beware of straightening your legs for a long rest between reps.

Visualization

Imagine you had a pile of $100 bills just under your buttocks. Every time you lower yourself, grab one with your buttocks! Hold on tight as you lift and don't drop it until you begin the next lowering rep. Try doing negatives holding the $100 bill as well.

REMINDERS:

1. Keep torso upright
2. "Sit back" into hips
3. Lift only halfway up
4. Press into heels

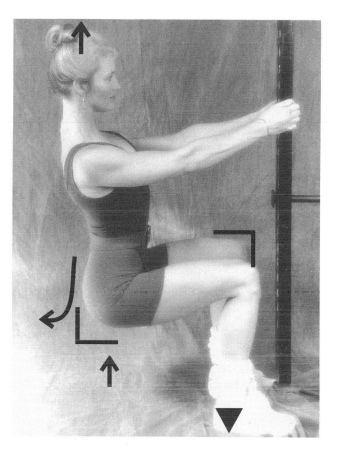

Variation The same movement can be done on a Smith Machine, a bar that slides on two poles. Depending on the machine, these bars can be quite light, with a "floating" effect. (Be careful, however, of the old, heavy Smith Machines with bars that weigh approximately 55 lbs.) In the Smith, maintain the same vertical position. This movement is anatomically impossible to do with a free bar on your back. Also try varying your foot position—feet together or hip-width apart. If you have trouble getting a full range of motion, try a *slightly* turned out wider stance. No full ballet turn-outs here—too risky on the knees. Keep your knees aligned over your ankles.

Leg Exercises

Exercise 3   Lunges

BASIC EXERCISE— with variations

The basic step-forward, step-back lunge is a tough exercise to do properly. Most people wobble side to side, lean forward in the torso, bang the back knee on the floor or step forward with so much force it stresses the front knee. For all that trouble, it doesn't get you much. The following variations are safer, more effective alternatives. Beginners need no additional weight. More advanced trainers should try these lunges in a Smith Machine or holding dumbbells. A heavy barbell on your shoulders tends to exacerbate any spine instability. A light bar or pole on your back, however, can give you a feeling of balance—as if balancing on a high wire.

Movement variations

For all versions of a lunge, place both hands on the front knee for more stability (if not holding a weight) or hold onto a railing or an upright broomstick for better balance.

Step-back lunges. Instead of stepping forward, step back 2 to 3 feet, keeping your torso upright (this eliminates forward force on the knee). As you bring your feet together, press your weight into the front *heel* for balance and extra "glute" awareness. Alternating legs gives each leg double rest time and is easier. Doing one leg only is obviously harder. It's your choice.

In-place lunges. Get yourself into a proper long stance before starting. Align your hips directly under your shoulders, with the front knee above or *behind* the ankle, and keep your back heel up. Stance is 2 to 3 feet long, hip-width wide and parallel. Lower down and lift. This can only be done one leg at a time.

Front leg elevated. (No more than 8 inches.) I recommend this advanced move for in-place lunges only. It *is* safe to lower your thigh below parallel *only* if your front knee is behind your heel. This way you still don't exceed a 90-degree angle in the knee—yet you go deeper to really tax the buttocks.

Back leg elevated. (Again no more than 8 inches—and again, keep the front knee over or behind your heel.) This puts more stress on the thigh of your back leg. A good pre-ski season exercise, this can also uncomfortably stretch out your hip flexor. After each set, stand or lie on the ground, pull your knee up to your chest and let it relax.

Drawing with the weight

Again, your spine is the weight you're lifting. Try to align the hip bone, lower back and shoulder in a vertical line.

Safety tips

Make sure your spine stays upright. This exercise takes a lot of control, so ease into it. Try going slow at first and/or stepping halfway back before doing the full step-back lunge. Also try moving just halfway down at first to "test the waters"

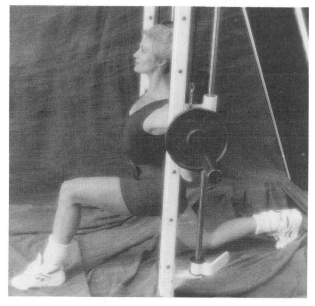

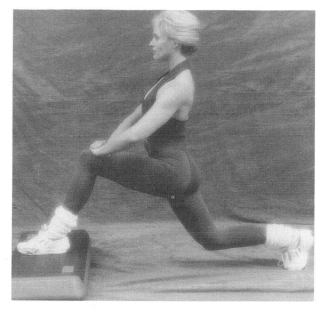

REMINDERS:

1. Keep torso vertical
2. Press heel into floor as you lift
3. Knee above or behind ankle

REMINDER:

1. Knee *behind* ankle when foot is elevated

in the in-place lunge. Keep your front knee *over* or slightly *behind* the ankle—not out over the toe. Hold in your abdominals to maintain the proper posture.

Targeted muscles	Quadriceps and gluteus on the front leg, quadriceps on the back leg. There's more buttocks involvement when the stance is longer, lunges are deeper and when the front foot is elevated.
Main moving joints	Knees and hips.
Function	Lunges help develop balance in hip stabilizing muscles as well as giving stride power and leg strength for walking, running and other athletics.
Aesthetics	Again, when these muscles are strengthened, the result is a pleasing roundness in the buttocks, shape and tone in the thigh.
Tricks of the trade	Lengthen the hip flexor on your back leg to better maintain posture.
No cheating	Beware of going so fast you're propelled by momentum.
Visualization	Imagine your torso is inside a narrow cylinder. Try lifting and lowering without touching the inside cylindrical walls.

Leg Exercises

Exercise 4   Leg Extension with Machine and Ankle Weights

BASIC EXERCISE

There has been much debate by exercise specialists about the value of this exercise. Some argue that this movement has no functional merit, since most of us, except soccer players, goal kickers and dancers don't do this action in real life. (Many sports physiologists prefer so-called "closed-chain" exercises where feet make contact with the floor or a platform.) Others argue that it's helpful in knee rehabilitation and general fitness since it strengthens the muscles around the knee, which are used in all types of motions. I believe it has value for this reason, and it isolates the quadriceps.

Movement

Sit upright in the chair of the leg extension machine, *gently* holding the handles. Foot pads should sit firmly on your ankles—not on your feet or shins. Your knees should bend just off the edge of the seat. Extend your legs without jamming your knees, and control the weight as you lower. Avoid bending your knee back beyond 90 degrees, as this can stress ligaments—especially with heavy weight.

With ankle weights

Sit on a bench or chair, placing one foot on the floor for better back support. Work one leg at a time.

Drawing with the weight

Lift the weight only from a 6 o'clock position to 9 o'clock or just below. Avoid taking it back to 5 o'clock.

Safety tips

Do not mimic those you might see who use heavy weight, dance around on the seat, go through a small r.o.m. (range of motion) and bang the plates between reps. Go slowly into that good pain.

Targeted muscles

Quads and quads alone.

Main moving joint

Knee—isolation exercise.

Function

A functional exercise for anyone who needs power in a forward kick. Also good for women with wide pelvises—helps strengthen the muscles surrounding the knees, thus reducing the stress on the knee caused by angled thigh bones.

Aesthetics

Gives shape and tone to the front of the thighs.

Tricks of the trade

I sometimes use my lifting belt to strap myself into the machine (however, this only works with a Velcro closure). Slide the buckle around one handle, tighten the Velcro end around the other handle and secure—especially valuable when using heavier weight.

Leg Exercises

REMINDERS:

1. Avoid "dead zone"
2. Keep buttocks on seat
3. Don't "jam" knees when legs straighten

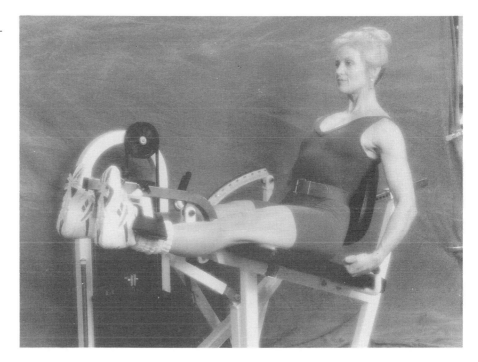

No cheating Try to keep your back completely still throughout the motion. Avoid unconsciously rotating your thighs in the hip sockets, as this displaces the workload. Keep buttocks on the seat!

Visualization Imagine your thigh muscles are giant sponges—wring out water with every rep.

Variation Rotating your toes inward about 45 degrees involves the "outer quads" more and rotating your toes outward, on the same angle, works the quads closer to the inside of the leg. However, don't do this if it bothers your knees. Stay parallel, and you work them all. Also, many machines have a lever arm that attaches to the side rather than the center of the machine. Thus, the leg closer to that lever ends up with a leverage advantage. Do one leg at a time to build equal strength in both legs.

Leg Exercises

Exercise 5   Hack Squat

INTERMEDIATE EXERCISE   Some old hack squat machines have heavy sliding pads that weigh about 45 lbs. even without plates. Newer versions are lighter and better for beginners. Hack squats let you work front and inner thighs and some gluteus much the way a squat does. However, because you're on a slant and guided by the hack squat machine, there isn't as much spinal compression as there is vertically with a bar on your back.

Movement   Place your feet at the far end of the foot rest, so your knees bend in a 90-degree angle. Many people find a hip-width stance with a *slight* turn-out allows greater r.o.m. Keep your back in neutral, not pelvic tilted. Release the safety handles and lower the weight. Use a weight that allows a full range of motion. Push up just short of straight, pressing into your *heels*.

Drawing with the weight   At the bottom of the motion, "draw" 90-degree angles with both hips and knees.

Safety tips   Make sure your spine stays neutral, your heels stay on the foot plate, your knees stay over your ankles—and avoid "dropping" down into your knees.

Targeted muscles   Front and inner thigh. Some buttocks involvement.

Main moving joints   Hips and knees.

Function   Basic leg strength. A good power move for all sorts of athletics.

Aesthetics   A shapely sweep to the thigh.

Tricks of the trade   If you have the strength to control it, you can safely lower your buttocks slightly *below* the hips to include more buttocks work. Just make sure your feet are far forward.

No cheating   Beware of bouncing through your reps. Also be careful not to arch or flatten your back.

Visualization   Imagine that with every rep, you "dip your butt in a bucket." As you lift, internally squeeze your thigh muscles, as if you're pulling up a pair of support stockings. Also, remember the pile of $100 bills? Pick one up in your cheeks with every lift.

REMINDERS:

1. Put feet at edge of platform
2. Knees and hips form 90-degree angles
3. Press into heels

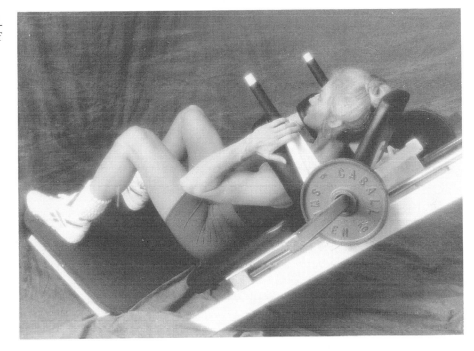

Variation Many people vary their foot positions to work different parts of the thigh—using a narrow stance for inner thigh and a wide stance for the outer thigh. Whether this really works is debatable. However, you might try different stances to see how they affect your balance.

For an advanced version of a hack squat, try using one leg at a time. Balance lightly on the other foot. Use no weight at first. Your r.o.m. will most likely be smaller by a third.

Leg Exercises

Exercise 6   Reverse Hack Squat

ADVANCED EXERCISE This is a more esoteric exercise, not recommended for beginners or anyone with any kind of back problems. It's yet another version of a squat, this time with the torso horizontal, facing down. Since the pad slides on an angle, this movement doesn't put direct vertical pressure on the spine (the back moves off the line of force). It doesn't bother my scoliosis and it certainly localizes the work in the buttocks!

Movement Stand backwards in a hack squat machine, with the pads on your shoulders and your heels halfway up the plate, so that when you bend your knees, your back ends up *parallel* to the floor. (You may have to experiment to find the most comfortable position.) Come up only three quarters of the way, without pressing your hips forward or changing your back position. This way you do all the pushing with your legs and the spine doesn't wobble.

Drawing with the weight As you lower, "draw" your back in a parallel line to the floor, with hips and knees in a 90-degree angle. At the top, try to maintain the same back position.

Safety tips Use weight that's light enough to handle so you don't feel the compression on your spine. Also, be careful not to jam your forehead into the pad and thus tense your neck and shoulder muscles. Press your hands into the pad for extra support.

Targeted muscles Buttocks, some quads.

Main moving joints Hips and knees.

Function Like other squats, this gives you overall leg power, with particular emphasis on the buttocks—good for climbing, dancing, sports that use running and jumping.

Aesthetics Tight, firm, rounded buttocks!

Tricks of the trade If you need a little more r.o.m., turn your feet out slightly, using a hip-width stance.

No cheating Be careful not to come up to a lock-kneed, resting stance between each rep.

Visualization Once again, grab the money at the bottom of each repetition. Drop it only as you lower.

Leg Exercises

REMINDERS:

1. Keep back parallel to floor, spine neutral

2. Avoid pushing hips forward as you come up

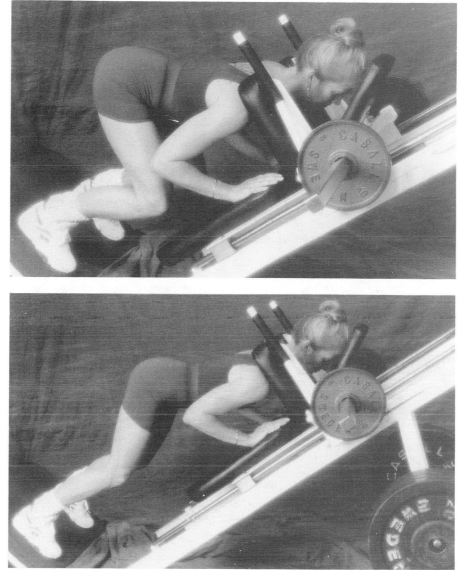

Variation For a humbling experience, try one leg at a time (rest the other foot gently on the plate for support). Use no weight at first. Be careful not to push your hip out to the side as you lower. If you can't see yourself, have someone watch to make sure you don't.

Leg Exercises

Exercise 7 "Stiff" Legged Deadlifts

VERY ADVANCED EXERCISE

This exercise requires finely tuned body awareness to do it right—most of the time it's done wrong. The secret is in maintaining a "flat" back position. No banana backs! Rounding forward not only shifts all the weight into the ligaments, discs and connective tissue of your spine, but also puts you at risk for overstretching hamstrings, which could cause injury there, too. However, done correctly, this is an excellent exercise for hamstrings and glutes.

"Stiff" legged doesn't mean the knees are locked straight—but that they are held in a soft, slightly bent position throughout and the angle doesn't change. (A regular deadlift uses bent knees and is a powerlifting move, similar to squats. It's a multi-muscle move for back and legs.)

Some people like to do stiff legged deadlifts standing on a block, to take the bar below the platform for a full stretch in the hamstrings. Most people can't stretch that far forward without bending the spine.

Use a barbell, dumbbells or the Smith Machine (my favorite—in it I feel more balanced). On the Smith, however, you have to stand on a bench because most of the machines have safety stops that keep the bar from sliding to the floor—thus limiting r.o.m.

Movement

Holding a bar or dumbbells, stand up straight, pull in your abs, and "puff" out your chest—which helps maintain a "flat" back. (The spine isn't actually flat, but in its natural curve.) Go only as far forward as your flat back will allow; the weights usually stop at shin level. "Slide" the bar or dumbbells down along your legs, close to your body. At the bottom of the motion, "sit back" into your hips to shift the weight into your heels—and therefore into your hips. Lift the bar only three quarters of the way, so the "force" stays with your hamstrings. Higher is a dead zone for hamstrings and involves much of the lower back.

Drawing with the weight

This is primarily a one-joint move at the hips, so technically it's an arcing motion. You might not see it at first, since the weight itself doesn't draw an arc—your *head* does. Although the motion starts with your head at 12 o'clock, the working part of the exercise starts with your head at 11 or 10 and ends at 9 o'clock or less, depending on your flexibility.

Safety

At every step along the way, be aware of your spine. Exaggerate pressing your chest forward and pulling in your abdominals to maintain form. Also, beware of swinging the free weight way out in front of your legs. To protect your neck muscles, tuck your chin under and look directly at the floor.

Targeted muscles

Hamstrings and glutes.

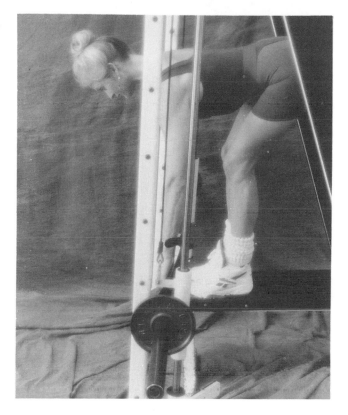

Main moving joint	Hips.
Function	In the world of aerobic dance, forward flexion has become a dirty word. However, forward flexion as done here doesn't tax the spine so much—since the muscles are *contracted*, therefore protected. It's when we're stretched and twisted or bouncing that we get into trouble. If you want to pick up a heavy box, don't use the form from this deadlift, but the bent-kneed, powerlifting deadlift, which is like a squat. The main difference is you pick up "dead" weight from the floor.
Aesthetics	This exercise targets where the back of the thigh meets the buttocks.
Tricks of the trade	In the full-stretch position, carefully lengthen your hamstrings (imagine they could stretch up and over your hip bones). Before you lift, squeeze your buttocks together, *then* come up.
No cheating	Don't round your back for more r.o.m.
Visualization	Imagine you're a robot with only one moving part—hips.

Leg Exercises

Exercise 8   Inner Thigh with Machine, Cables and Ankle Weights

BASIC EXERCISE This exercise isolates the inner thigh muscles (or adductors). Since the adductors already work hard during squats and lunges, it's a good idea to do one of these complementary exercises on the same day you do the others.

Movement For this exercise you'll use the seated adductor machine: Unfortunately many such machines have slanted seats that make you lean back. If the seat's adjustable, bring it upright. If not, you can place an extra pad behind the back for greater lower back support. Sitting upright lets you support the torso with abdominal strength and gives better inner thigh isolation, makes the exercise feel harder with less weight. Slowly squeeze the legs together, hold and open with control. Don't bang the plates.

With cables Some cable machines feel heavier than others, depending on how many round pulleys there are per cable. More pulleys = more leverage = lighter weight. Use cables only if you can use 5 lbs. or less. Place a bench between two cables. Put a cuff around each ankle and attach the cable with a clip. Lie back on the bench and start by bringing your feet together (so your first move is a "lower"). Then carefully open your legs and lift again, but only halfway up, to keep constant tension on the muscle. Work with slightly bent knees.

With ankle weights It's the same motion as with cables.

Drawing with the weight On the machine, you set the r.o.m. so your left leg starts at 10 o'clock and your right leg at 2 o'clock. Both legs meet at 12 o'clock. However, with cables, bring your legs only halfway together—going from 10 to 11 on your left leg and 2 to 1 on your right leg. Taking your legs up to 12 o'clock removes resistance and puts you in the "dead zone."

Safety tips Beware of overstretching your inner thigh on any of these. Be sure that the resistance isn't so heavy that it pulls your legs apart.

Targeted muscles Inner thighs (or adductors).

Main moving joint Hip (top of thigh bone, moving in hip socket). Don't add knees.

Function Any time you squeeze your thighs together, you use this motion. It's also used in many sports—riding a horse, the lateral motions of tennis, soccer, dancing.

Aesthetics Firm inner thighs!

Leg Exercises

REMINDERS:

1. Use only 5 lbs. or less

2. Lift legs halfway up to avoid "dead zone"

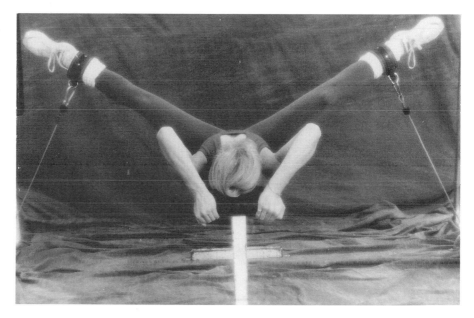

Tricks of the trade Use pointed toes to make this more challenging, flexed feet to make it easier.

No cheating It's imperative that you don't bounce through your stretch, or you could easily pull a muscle.

Visualization Imagine you have a giant beach ball between your legs—squeeze it.

Variation Try this turned out and parallel. Also experiment with slow, controlled pulses at various parts of the motion.

Leg Exercises

Exercise 9   Hip Extension with Cables and Ankle Weights

BASIC EXERCISE   Forget those old-fashioned leg swings (with the back arching out of control). This exercise is best performed slowly, in a shorter r.o.m. The key to effectiveness is making sure your spine remains stable.

Movement   With ankle cuff attached to floor cable. Align the bench so the narrow end faces the cable. Also move the bench just off center to the pulley, so your working leg can lift directly away from the fixed point (not on an angle). Put on an ankle cuff and clip it to the cable. Kneel on the bench, with one knee. Use both hands to balance, keeping your back parallel to the floor. Your working leg hangs down so your foot just misses the floor. Movement starts with the knee slightly bent, and ends with your leg straight in line with your spine—but think of this as a one-joint move.

With ankle weights   Perform the same motion, as above.

Drawing with the weight   Start with your working foot in the 6 o'clock position (even though your knee might be closer to 7 o'clock) and lift it to 3 o'clock.

Safety tips   Keep your back completely still throughout the movement. Don't raise your leg above the 3 o'clock position—it's too tempting to arch the back. And beware of leaning into the supporting hip.

Main moving joint   Focus on the hip joint only. Your knee plays a secondary role, preventing your leg from touching the floor.

Function   Good for developing "push-off" strength, as when you climb hills.

Aesthetics   High, rounded, gravity-defying buttocks!

Tricks of the trade   Balance on the "inside" of the supporting knee so your weight stays centered.

No cheating   No momentum, no swinging leg.

Visualization   Imagine your hip is the hub of a wheel.

Variation   Try this with pointed feet to make the exercise more difficult—with less assistance from calves. Also, try a slight turn-out, as in ballet, to address the buttocks muscles from a different angle.

Leg Exercises

REMINDERS:

1. Hip (not knee) is main joint
2. Hold torso steady

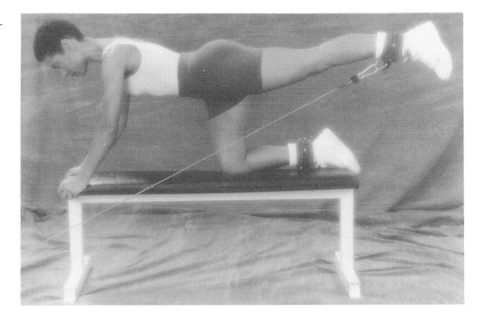

Leg Exercises

Exercise 10   Multi-Hip Machine

BASIC EXERCISE This is a popular machine in most gyms and is often used to tone up the old buttocks. But bad form tends to reign supreme. The tendency is to swing the leg and spine—and, thus, bypass the benefits. This machine also has three adjustable parts—so it takes patience to find the best position. Despite its problems, this exercise still has value.

Movement Stand up so that your spine is *vertical* and the supporting knee is slightly bent. To make it a little easier on your back, you can incline your torso forward *from the hips*, about 5 to 15 degrees—but avoid rounding the lower back. Position the rolling pad just under your knee. Press your thighs backwards.

Drawing with the weight Technically, this is a circular motion because it's primarily a one-joint move. It's your *thigh* (not your shin) that traces the hands of a clock face, starting at 7 o'clock and ending at 4.

Safety tips Beware of bringing your knee so far forward that it causes your back to round—or so far back that you arch.

Targeted muscles Gluteus muscles.

Main moving joint Hip. Knee moves slightly.

Function In life, we don't do this movement too often. Yet strengthened glutes assist in all sorts of motions—climbing, running, jumping, dancing . . .

Aesthetics This exercise is done more for form than function. Again, it's a butt-tightener and lifter.

Tricks of the trade To keep proper form, keep your shin parallel to the floor throughout.

No cheating Lots of people use heavy weight and wildly swing out of control. Don't be one of them. Make sure you hold each contraction and keep your spine upright.

Visualization As you press your leg back, flex your foot and imagine you're putting your footprint on the wall behind you. This gives you more control and therefore more buttocks work.

Variation Try small, controlled pulses at various steps along the way.

Leg Exercises

REMINDERS:

1. Keep torso still and upright
2. Use a small r.o.m.

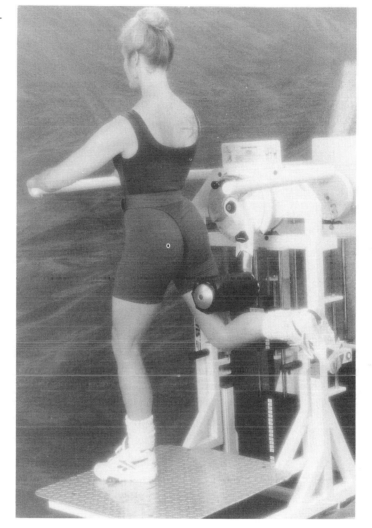

Leg Exercises

Exercise 11 Standing Hamstring Curls with Machine and Ankle Weights

BASIC EXERCISE—using ankle weights INTERMEDIATE EXERCISE—using the machine

Hamstrings don't get as much action as quads in squats, lunges and leg presses: They respond best to isolation work. This exercise is a very effective hamstring strengthener, since it works in a vertical position, directly against gravity. Done with correct form, the muscle doesn't need much resistance to reach fatigue.

Movement

Standing hamstring curl machine. Stand with your body in a pure vertical (no bending forward at the waist or hips). Elevate the supporting foot slightly (i.e., stand on a 10-lb. plate or a 2-by-4), so your working foot doesn't hit the floor. Keep your knees next to each other, so the thigh doesn't move back or forward (thus adding the hip joint). Simply curl the heel of your working leg toward your buttocks, squeeze the muscle at the top and lower with control. Use very light weight at first. Using weight that's too heavy will tempt you to incline your torso and stick out your butt.

With ankle weight

For extra balance, hold on to something. Raise heels to buttocks, as above.

Drawing with the weight

Again, this is a one-joint, arcing move. Start with your foot at 6 o'clock, stop at 2 o'clock, lower all the way.

Safety tips

Keep your back and hips still—the only moving part is your lower leg. Slightly bend the supporting knee and beware of sticking out your butt!

Targeted muscles

Hamstrings.

Main moving joint

Knee. Some people like to add a hip extension (thigh lifting backwards) for more contraction in gluteus muscles. However, this often results in arching the lower back. Keep it a one-joint move for better isolation of your hamstrings.

Function

Hamstrings add stability for the entire lower body—and also provide a firm foundation to posture (weak hamstrings can contribute to spinal misalignment and lower back pain, too). This is a much-neglected muscle.

Aesthetics

A developed hamstring adds a sexy sweep to the backside of the leg, giving a round, full appearance. Once you get used to seeing developed hamstrings, a leg without them will look like something's missing!

REMINDERS:

1. Keep spine vertical

2. Knee is the only moving joint

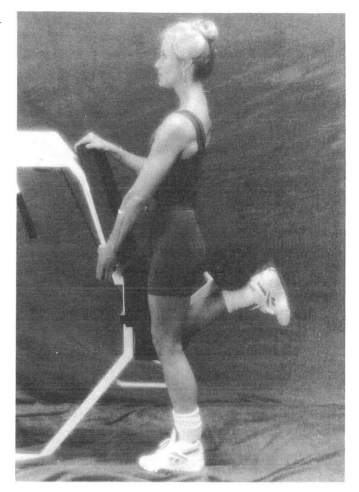

Tricks of the trade   Press hips ever so slightly forward to lengthen your hip flexor as you do the move. Also squeeze your buttocks. These two actions give you much better control. Just be careful not to overstretch the hip flexors and arch the back. Try adding pulses at the lower, middle and upper parts of the move.

No cheating   No momentum, no whacking up the weight. Avoid going beyond 2 o'clock, up into the dead zone.

Visualization   Once again, imagine squeezing that $100 bill between your buttocks as you do the movement and keep the squeeze as you lower your leg.

Variation   Point your toes to minimize assistance from your calves.

Leg Exercises

Exercise 12   Prone Hamstring Curl

BASIC EXERCISE   This exercise supports the torso—but don't be fooled. It's still easy to cheat by raising the hips—adding another joint, more muscles and hyperextension of the lower back.

Movement   Position yourself on the prone hamstring curl machine so the bend in the pad touches the top of your hip bones. (If you have an old-fashioned flat pad, place a small, rolled-up towel under your hips.) Push your pelvis into the pad. Lightly hold on to the handles. Lift your feet three quarters of the way up.

Drawing with the weight or band   Using the clock face, you might feel disoriented in this position since your body is pitched forward. It's easier to imagine that your *feet* point to 6 o'clock, then lift to 10 o'clock.

Safety tips   Press your hips down, down, down into the pad for more spinal stability and better hamstring isolation. Beware not to jerk up the weight (and hit yourself in the buttocks with the bar) or raise your thighs. Also, keep the back of the neck long, not arched, throughout, and avoid white-knuckling the handles.

Targeted muscles   Hamstrings.

Main moving joint   Knees.

Function   Again, developed hamstrings add stability for the lower body and torso, lend strength and performance ability for sports.

Aesthetics   Strengthened hamstrings create a curve where once there was a line—definition where there was none.

Tricks of the trade   To make it harder to cheat, raise your spine off the pad so it's parallel to the floor (but not arched). To involve the buttocks more as stabilizers, squeeze them together not only as you lift (squeeze that well-worn $100 bill), but keep the squeeze as you slowly lower.

No cheating   No weight hurling or plate banging, no backs arching or butts lifting to the sky.

Visualization   Imagine that a large person is sitting on your hips and there's no way you can lift him or her.

Variation   Try one leg at a time for better controlled isolation and a more "honest" exercise (devoid of the advantage "bought" with two legs). This is also a good place to do "21's"—7 small reps in just the lower half of the move, 7 small reps in just the upper half of the move, followed by 7 reps throughout the full r.o.m. Whew!

Leg Exercises

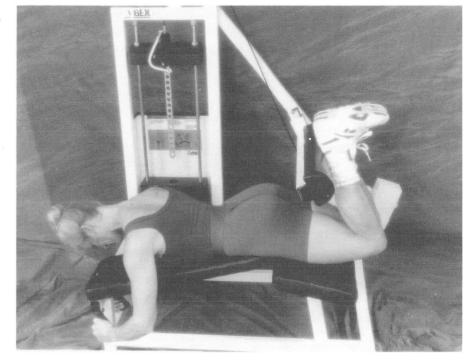

Leg Exercises

Exercise 13 Leg Raises with No Weight or Ankle Weight

BASIC EXERCISE Contrary to popular belief, this exercise doesn't work the thighs, but a small muscle on the outer hip called the tensor fasciae latae. This is a hip stabilizer—very important for balance and a good preventive against injury when you're doing other exercises like lunges.

Movement For a fuller r.o.m., lie on a decline bench or step. Rest your arm over the edge. Bend your bottom knee at a 45-degree angle to balance the torso. Align your pelvis so the top hip bone rests directly above the lower—i.e., don't lean back. Keep your leg parallel (don't turn out at the hip to get the leg higher—that eliminates the working muscle). Lift your leg only as high as you can without losing form.

With ankle weight Same motion as above using 1-to-5-lb. weights (5 lbs. feels very heavy!).

Drawing with the weight This one-joint, arcing motion starts at 8 o'clock and lifts to 10 o'clock. If you can't reach 10, at least lift to 9.

Safety tips Be careful not to lean the top shoulder back. Use your abdominal strength to hold your position. Lift and lower your leg with control.

Targeted muscles Tensor fasciae.

Main moving joint Hip joint.

Function Balance for walking, running, climbing, dancing and doing lunges.

Aesthetics When this muscle is developed it creates a gentle, beautiful indentation along the hip, sometimes called "the dancer's dimple."

Tricks of the trade The greater r.o.m. achieved on the decline bench makes this exercise much more valuable and challenging than on a flat floor.

No cheating No turning out your leg as you lift. No leaning back.

Visualization Imagine you have a piece of chalk between your toes. Draw that arc in the same place every time. Also, reach "out and up," with your leg lengthening at the hip joint with each lift.

Variation Try different angles of the leg—keep it in line with the spine or angle your leg forward to 45 degrees. To include the gluteus medius muscle a bit more, rotate your leg in the hip socket and angle your toe towards the ground.

REMINDERS:

1. Keep top hip bone directly over lower

2. Bend bottom knee for support, soften top knee

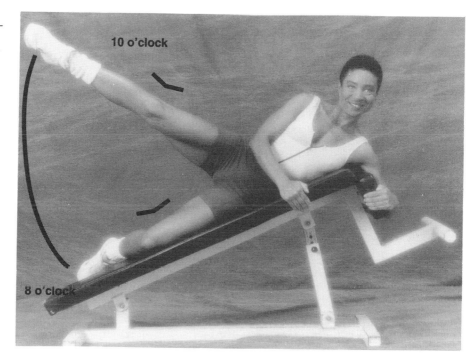

10 o'clock

8 o'clock

Calf Exercises

Exercise 14 Toe Press on Leg Press Machine

BASIC EXERCISE Calves are among the toughest muscles to "grow." They're the second most densely woven muscles in the body (after the jaw). They have to be tough so you can walk on them all day. Genetics play a big part in calf size. It seems you've either got 'em or you don't. If you don't, you can make them stronger and, yes, a bit bigger and more shapely, but don't expect miracles. (That's why plastic surgeons invented calf implants.) Calves consist of two muscles—the surface, bulbous "diamond shaped" gastrocnemius, which adds muscle shape, and the more subtle, deeply hidden soleus, which contributes more to muscle size. This one's for the "gastroc."

Movement Use the Leg Press machine as in Exercise 1. Place the balls of your feet on the *bottom* of the foot plate this time. Press toes all the way forward and all the way back in a full r.o.m. (you may or may not need to release the safety handles, depending on your leg length). Keep your knees "soft." I prefer this exercise to standing calf work because you can use a lot of weight without having it bear down on your spine.

Drawing with the weight Toes travel from about 11 o'clock to 2 o'clock.

Safety tips Beware of locking out your legs (it's stressful for the ligaments).

Targeted muscle Gastrocnemius.

Main moving joint Ankle.

Function Walking, running, dancing, skipping, jumping around—can't move without them!

Aesthetics High heels were invented to show off shapely calves. Yet, strong calves look just as good in flats. A well-shaped calf adds a finishing touch to the leg.

Tricks of the trade Get a "double squeeze." Go to the top of the contraction and squeeze—then go a millimeter higher and squeeze again, as if balancing on 6-inch heels. Do the same in reverse. Stretch and then stretch a bit further. Also, try occasional high-rep training—using 30 to 50 reps!

No cheating Avoid bouncing, or using little half-reps. Some folks will load every plate, sit their friends on top of the weight stack and then lift the whole thing about 1 inch—screaming all the way. This benefits the ego more than the calves.

Calf Exercises

REMINDERS:

1. Use a full stretch and a "double squeeze"
2. Keep knees soft

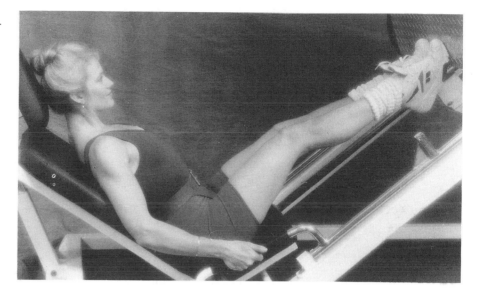

Visualization With each contraction of the calves, imagine your calves are the shape and size of tennis balls.

Variation A turned-out position works a bit more of the "outer head." A turned-in position, however, doesn't significantly target the "inner head."

Calf Exercises

Exercise 15   Seated Calf Raise

BASIC EXERCISE   The seated calf raise targets the soleus muscle—the deeper of the two calf muscles, responsible for size. When the knee is bent, the use of the gastrocnemius is minimal.

Movement   Sit in the seated calf machine—or on a bench, with your toes raised on a block with a barbell resting on your knees.

Drawing with the weight   Raise heels from 8 o'clock to 10 o'clock—more if you have the mobility.

Safety tips   Make sure you've got the balls of your feet firmly placed so they don't slip off the block.

Targeted muscle   Soleus.

Main moving joint   Ankle.

Function   The soleus lets you point and flex your feet! Strong calves help you in all "push-off" sports, such as tennis, dancing, volleyball and running.

Aesthetics   The soleus gives the calf size.

Tricks of the trade   Once again, go for the double squeeze. Squeeze once at the top of the motion, pull up a bit higher and squeeze again. Also, if your seat tilts back every time you raise heels, try countering the motion by slightly leaning your torso into each lift.

No cheating   Don't shorten the r.o.m. to lift more weight. Go for full reps.

Visualization   As you contract, pull your calves "up" inside your shins.

Variation   Try one leg at a time. Don't bother with toes in or toes out, as all positions virtually work the same.

Calf Exercises

REMINDER:

1. Use full r.o.m.

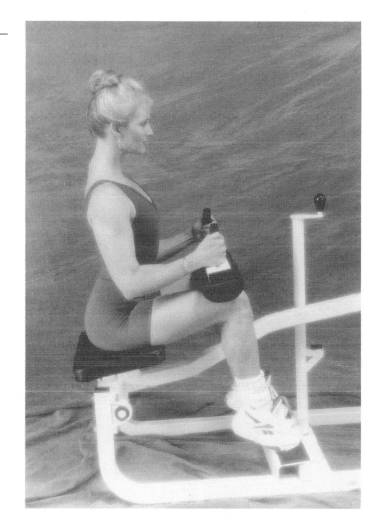

Calf Exercises

Exercise 16   Standing Calf Raise

BASIC EXERCISE   I like the simplicity and effectiveness of this exercise—sans equipment. Done one leg at a time, it also tests your balance and lets you work on bringing up your weaker side. (People who drive a car with a clutch often have a heftier left calf. People who drive a car with an automatic transmission have a bigger right one.)

Movement   Stand on one foot on an elevated block or stair. Soften your supporting knee. *Lightly* balance your body on a wall or pole in front of you. To add more resistance, hold onto one dumbbell. Push up onto the ball of your supporting foot, lifting your heel. What you're lifting here is your full body weight—balanced on just one calf. For better balance, slightly turn out your supporting foot. Repeat using the other leg.

Drawing with the weight   Again, your heel lifts from 4 to 2 o'clock—more if you have it!

Safety tips   Keep the supporting knee slightly bent.

Targeted muscles   Gastrocnemius and soleus.

Main moving joint   Ankle.

Function   Every motion that requires walking or running!

Aesthetics   This exercise combines gastroc and soleus work—thus it does double duty by enhancing both shape and size.

Tricks of the trade   Again, use the "double squeeze" technique.

No cheating   Don't lean into that wall or put too much weight into your supporting arm! Also make sure you press straight *up*, not off to one side.

Visualization   Imagine that you're standing in a very narrow cylinder. Press up and lower down without touching the inside walls.

Variation   Try this in a standing calf machine—one or two feet at a time.

REMINDER:

1. Push whole body up on a clean vertical line

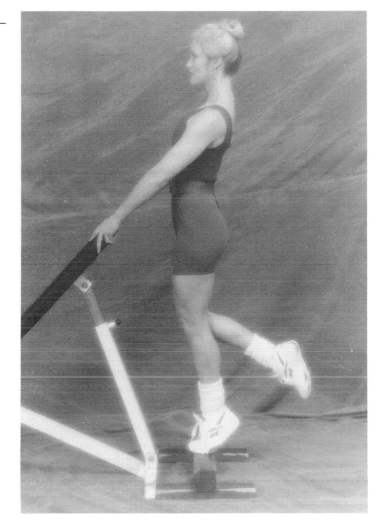

Back Exercises

Exercise 17   Pull-Downs to Chest

(**Note:** Many upper body moves are shown with a "thumbless grip"—a position that decreases the thumb's leverage advantage, and by default, helps you keep your wrists straight. Beginners, however, may feel more comfortable wrapping their thumbs around the bar.)

BASIC EXERCISE   The secret to all back exercises is to initiate the movement *from the back*. Sounds logical enough, but most people pull from the arms first and then round the back—which means the targeted muscles—the lats (latissimus dorsi)—can't even contract at all, and the arms do all the work! Proper form is essential so that this exercise is not a waste of time. The pull-down to the chest puts less rotational strain on shoulders than a pull-down behind the neck. Less weight is needed, too, for the exercise to be effective. If you have no shoulder problems, a pull-down behind the neck is fine (try slightly inclining the torso forward, yet holding it still for a more stable spine).

Movement   On the Pull-down machine, take an overhand grip on a long angled bar, with your hands right on the "bend" or slightly wider. Sit up very tall, so that when you pull down the bar, it safely clears your nose! (You may have to sit back on an extra bench, slightly behind the allotted seat.) Imagine that your arms seem to attach to your waist. 1) Shrug your shoulders *down*; i.e., "engage or depress the scapula," but don't bend your arms just yet. 2) *Then* add the arms. Focus on lifting your chest to meet the bar, rather than collapsing your chest. *Arch your upper back* and support your lower back with abdominals held strong. 3) Straighten your arms, being careful not to overstretch your shoulders. 4) Stretch your lats by letting your shoulders shrug up slightly. At first, make it a point to differentiate between each move. As you become more seasoned, let the moves flow into one another.

Drawing with the weight   This is a multi-joint move. Be conscious of "drawing" a straight horizontal line with the bar—pull evenly. Get your elbows behind your back.

Safety tips   Beware of adding a swing in the lower back to lift more weight. This lets you cheat with heavier weight—but doesn't let you "hold the squeeze," as it's harder to control the motion. Don't let the weights jerk up your shoulders. Use abdominal strength to keep your torso still and aligned.

Targeted muscles   Lats, rhomboids and teres muscles.

Main moving joints   Shoulders and elbows.

Function   This exercise is especially good at strengthening the "good posture muscles" in the upper back.

1. Pull back muscles first, then add arms
2. Lift chest to meet bar
3. Elbows go behind back

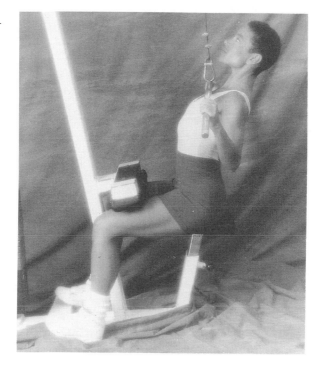

Aesthetics   We don't often get to see our backs. But strong, sleek back muscles give the torso a look of fine, chiseled sculpture. Developed lats help give the torso a flattering V shape, creating the illusion of a narrow waist.

Tricks of the trade   When doing seated pull-downs, keep your feet flat on the floor, with your knees at a 90-degree angle to better "ground" yourself. Press your heels into the floor for better stabilization. Also try sitting backwards on the seat, so you face out for a change. Without pads over your knees, you're forced to stabilize yourself—and can't cheat.

No cheating   No slumping, no arching the lower spine, no rocking on the tailbone.

Visualization   As you lift your chest to meet the bar, think of the bowsprit mermaids that adorn the bows of old sailing ships. Borrow their brave, open posture or imagine the posture of a swan dive. Also, as the bar meets your chest, "squeeze your wings together."

Variation   Experiment with different handles and grips. A wide grip, especially with a straight bar, is hardest. A narrow grip with a V handle rotates the palms and gives you more biceps assistance—making it easier to handle more weight. An underhand grip or bar with two handles on the end also allows the biceps to assist.

Back Exercises

Exercise 18   Straight Arm Pull-Downs

NOT SO BASIC— but an excellent back isolator
This back exercise removes the biceps completely—thus, it's all back work and could help wake up your back muscles if you've had trouble feeling them. Since you're working with straight arms and just the shoulder joint, you have to use lighter weight than on a regular pull-down, which uses two joints. It also takes a little experimentation to position yourself at a comfortable distance from the pulley.

Movement
On any overhead cable machine, use a palm-down grip on a rotating bar. Sit back slightly into bent knees and hips, so you counter your weight from the pulley. Start with your arms parallel to the floor and press the bar down to your thighs, then add an extra squeeze in the lats (just under your armpits). *Slowly* release.

Drawing with the weight
Start with your arms at 9 o'clock; take the bar to 6 o'clock—further if you straighten your legs a bit.

Safety tips
Keep your elbow joints soft—not locked or bending throughout. If this bothers your elbows, lighten the weight. Keep your wrists straight and use your abdominals to maintain proper alignment. Also avoid lifting your arms above 9 o'clock—it's too taxing on the shoulders.

Targeted muscles
Lats, teres, rear delts and a bit of the long head of the triceps.

Main moving joint
Shoulders.

Function
This is a good exercise for swimmers—especially freestylers—and tennis players, for the serve. It's not a very common exercise—but it is a valuable one for isolating back muscles. I use it as a warmup exercise on back day.

Aesthetics
A well-developed upper back and V taper in the torso.

Tricks of the trade
Sit back in your heels and pull in your abdominals with every press.

No cheating
It's especially important to use no momentum here, no "windup" swing to press down the weight—since so much work hinges on the shoulders.

Visualization
When you bring the weight down, "see" the back muscles contract in a V. Also, keep your upper arms close to or touching the torso.

Variation
Try this with a single handle for more r.o.m. Take your hand *behind* the thigh—stopping at 5 o'clock, rather than 6.

1. Sit back away from pulley and incline torso slightly to "counter" weight

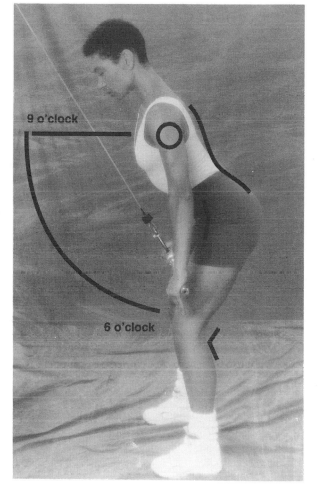

9 o'clock

6 o'clock

Back Exercises

Exercise 19 One-Arm Row with Dumbbell or Cable

BASIC EXERCISE The secrets of the one-arm row are these:

- Keep your back flat (in its natural curve), not hunched
- *Initiate the movement from the back* first, then add the arm (as with all back work)
- Keep your chest facing the floor, and your torso steady; don't twist
- Pull your elbow close to the hip (rather than the shoulder) for better control of your lat muscle; also kneel on a bench for support

Movement *With a dumbbell.* Start with the arm hanging straight down, on the direct line of gravity. As with the pull-down, 1) pull the upper back only, keeping your arm straight, 2) *then* pull up your elbow, 3) release your arm, 4) release your back muscles—without rounding.

With a cable. The advantage of the cable is that your line of force is on an oblique, not a vertical, so you can stretch forward and have resistance throughout a fuller r.o.m.

Drawing with the weight This is a two-joint move—thus, the weights trace a line. With a dumbbell, the line is almost vertical. With a cable, the line is more oblique—anywhere from 30 to 45 degrees, depending on how close you position yourself to the cable.

REMINDERS:

1. Initiate move from *back*, then add arms
2. Keep spine neutral
3. Pull elbow to hip

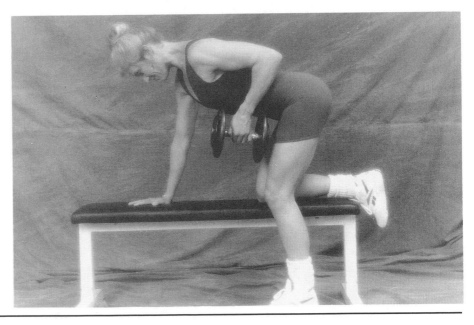

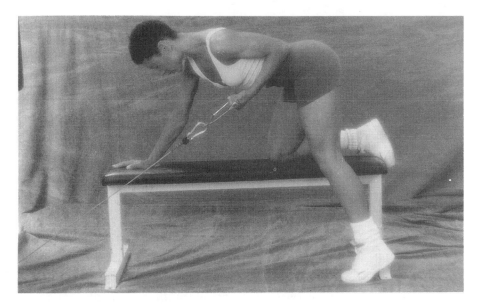

Safety tips	Be sure your back is supported and stays in neutral, with lower back muscles *contracted* throughout. Rounding your back will stretch muscles and therefore won't allow you to contract them. Also, beware of your hips shifting to one side and locking your supporting elbow.
Targeted muscles	Lats and rhomboids.
Main moving joints	Shoulder and elbow.
Function	This one helps build good core strength for lots of different movements. Working one side at a time is especially good for people with scoliosis—and in general, brings up a weaker side especially if you add a few more reps to that side. Also good for swimmers, rowers, tennis players, wind surfers.
Aesthetics	Good posture, V-tapered torso.
Tricks of the trade	The trick here is to keep it simple. Don't add funny rotations from the shoulder, or swing the dumbbell forward, trying to achieve more stretch. Keep your palm facing your body. At the top of the motion, squeeze your back muscles—and if you wish, rotate your palm up for a biceps squeeze. But, remember, this is a *back*, not an arm, exercise.
No cheating	Your back should remain still throughout—no twisting or lifting with momentum to jerk up a heavy weight.
Visualization	When kneeling on the bench, keep your back parallel to the floor (like a warped tabletop) or on a small, sloping angle, with your shoulders slightly above the hips.
Variation	With no bench handy, support yourself by holding onto *something*, so your torso is at least angled forward 45 degrees.

Back Exercises

Exercise 20   Seated Cable Row

BASIC EXERCISE   Once again, this back exercise uses a rowing motion. Thus, as before, it shouldn't be just an arm motion—but one that starts in the back and ends with a good back squeeze!

Movement   On a seated cable row machine sit with your torso upright, knees bent slightly, and make sure not to rock the lower back. 1) Squeeze your shoulders together, keeping your arms straight. 2) Pull your elbows behind your back. 3) Release your arms. 4) Release the lats—without rounding forward into the lower back or shoulders.

Drawing with the weight   Many machines let you vary the angle of pull on the cable, from low to high. Wherever that cable points, draws a straight line into the area of muscle that receives the most work.

Safety tips   Rounding forward for a "stretch" between reps not only compromises the lower back but also puts your shoulder rotator cuffs in a precarious position.

Targeted muscles   Lats and rhomboids.

Main moving joints   Shoulders and elbows—not your lower back!

Function   Strong back muscles assist in all pulling actions, general torso stability and in most sports!

Aesthetics   V-tapered torso, strong posture.

Tricks of the trade   Every time you pull in your arms, *push* your chest forward. When using a narrow grip, pull your elbows close to the torso.

No cheating   No yanking, bouncing or rounding forward or back.

Visualization   Imagine you could squeeze a pencil between your shoulder blades. Hold it there with every rep.

Variation   Use a single handle to isolate each side. Also, a wide grip on a straight bar will give you more upper back involvement. (Since upper back muscles are smaller, use less weight.) Also, if the machine allows, adjust the pulley so it comes from higher and lower angles.

Lower back variation   To add a lower back strengthener to the motion, incline your torso about 15 degrees forward (without rounding), then pull it upright. After that, complete the exercise as above.

Back Exercises

REMINDERS:

1. Sit upright
2. Pull back muscles first, *then* add arms
3. Lift chest to meet the bar

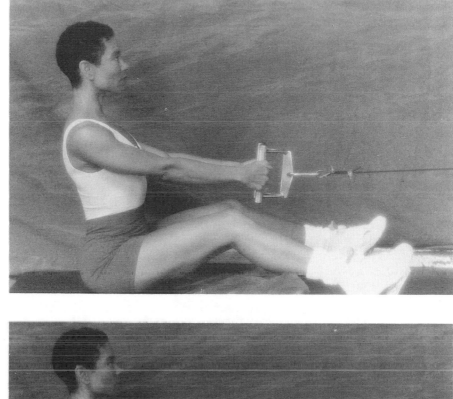

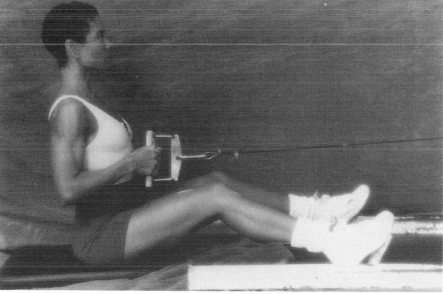

Back Exercises

Exercise 21　Lower Back Hyperextension

BASIC EXERCISE　Because of all the warnings about lower back safety, many people are actually *afraid* to work their lower backs—though these muscles need exercise, too. Many people do this exercise with the back hanging at a 90-degree angle, head pointing down. This angle can be uncomfortable for some, as it hangs all upper body weight off the lower vertebrae—which is hard on some people's discs. It also requires hip and glute involvement (there is a version of this exercise for glutes and hams—but it's hard to do well and isn't, in my opinion, the best exercise for those parts). Here, I prefer to curl and uncurl just the back, one vertebra at a time, as if doing an abdominal curl in reverse, to really target the lower back.

Movement　Anchor your body into the hyperextension bench, with your hips supported on a pad, and your feet secured. Avoid locking your knees if possible. Start in a flat-back position—with your torso parallel to the floor. Round your head, shoulders, upper back, middle and lower back down to a 45-degree position. Then, slowly reverse action to raise your spine back up to parallel or slightly above, if you have the mobility.

Drawing with the weight　Done slowly, this is a gentle arcing motion for the spine. Your head moves from 8 o'clock to 9 o'clock, more if you're flexible.

Safety tips　Be sure not to swing with momentum. Beware of overarching the spine.

Targeted muscles　Erector spinae.

Main moving joints　Spinal vertebrae—in lower and mid back.

Function　Builds strength in the lower back, thus preventing lower back pain caused by weakness.

Aesthetics　When lower back muscles are strong, they don't look showy like shoulders or biceps. However, they do help hold a firm posture, which is sexy indeed!

Tricks of the trade　Here, the best trick is to do it with care.

No cheating　It's tough to cheat on this if you minimize the momentum.

Visualization　See the lower back muscles as the "epicenter" of the motion. Curl and uncurl around it.

Variation　To add resistance, hold a 5-to-10-lb. plate at the chest.

Back Exercises

REMINDER:

1. Curl and uncurl spine as if doing an abdominal curl in reverse

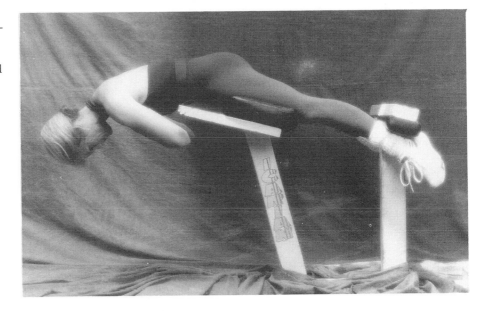

Chest Exercises

Exercise 22   Bench Press

BASIC EXERCISE   All chest exercises can be done in a flat, inclined or declined position, to focus on different parts of the fan-shaped pectoral muscle, though each exercise also works all parts, to different degrees. A flat bench targets the center part of the chest (which is good for overall strength), an incline targets the upper chest (elongating the cleavage) and a decline targets the lower chest. Chest muscles are strongest on a decline, next strongest on flat, and third strongest on an incline (because there's more meat on the lower portion of the pecs). Some argue that women don't need decline work, since that part of the muscle is covered with breast tissue but, since the lower portion has muscle, too, it also needs attention—plus, it's satisfying to be able to press more weight in this position. It's also possible to get a good pump throughout the whole chest with a decline. However, flat and incline are more common for women and yield more visible results.

Movement   (Use a free bar or Smith Machine) Lie on a bench and put your feet on the floor—not on the bench: This keeps the spine in neutral and creates more stability—it makes you use your abdominals, too. If pressing a heavy free weight, be sure to use a spotter. Balance the bar directly over the targeted part of your muscle (at the nipple line for a flat bench, just above your breasts for an incline, just below the nipple line for a decline). Lower the bar so it gently touches, but doesn't bounce off, your chest. Just beware this doesn't hurt your shoulders. If it does, only lower within your pain-free r.o.m. *Keep your chest lifted as you press the bar up!*

With dumbbells: It's more comfortable on your shoulder rotators if your thumbs rotate up towards your face—either at a 45- or a 90-degree angle (as opposed to thumbs pointing towards each other). Press the weights together in an A shape, keeping your pecs lifted to the ceiling as you straighten your arms.

Drawing with the weight   When using a bar, hold it wide enough so that your forearms are perpendicular to the floor when your arms bend (the same is true for dumbbells). If you use an Olympic bar, try putting your middle or ring finger on the bar's "groove." (An Olympic bar is the traditional long barbell used for Olympic-style and power lifts. Unloaded, it weighs 45 pounds.) Make sure your bar stays straight—no dipping to one side, no "torquing" or rotating (a spotter can let you know). With dumbbells, press the weights in a clean A shape, though they needn't bang together at the top.

Safety tip   Contrary to what some may tell you, don't "lock out" your elbows or throw your shoulders forward. These actions not only jar joints and tendons, but cause chest muscles to concave. Be sure to keep your hips on the bench and your back still.

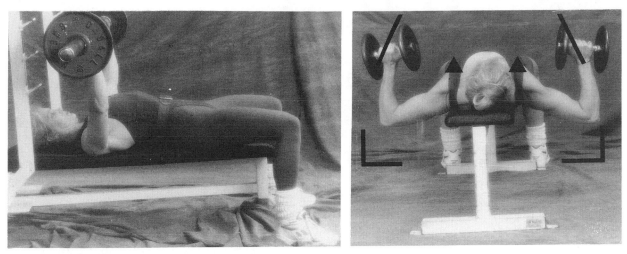

REMINDERS:

1. Keep spine neutral, hips down

2. Avoid "dropping" weights as you lower

3. Avoid locking elbows or throwing shoulders forward when you lift

4. Lift chest more as you press the weight

Targeted muscles	Center part of the chest and the front shoulder muscle. Triceps also assist.
Main moving joints	Shoulders and elbows.
Function	This helps with all pressing or pushing motions—the core of our frontal upper body strength.
Aesthetics	Developed upper chest muscles give the chest area a healthy roundness, definition, cleavage and they help hold up the breasts!
Tricks of the trade	Rest your feet gently on the floor. As the work gets harder, press your heels into the floor (keeping your hips down) to give you a leverage advantage reserve. With light weight, try "stops," resting the bar on your chest for half a second—then press "dead weight." Or try half-reps, lifting the bar only halfway up.
No cheating	No momentum, no hip lifting, back arching, shoulder throwing or elbow locking.
Visualization	With every rep, let the pectorals thrust into each other.
Variations	Use different angled benches (for inclines a 45-degree angled bench works best; higher angle than that works the shoulders). Alternate dumbbells, barbells, cables as well as machine presses if you have the equipment. Also, a wider grip on the bar targets the outer portion of the muscle—yet is harder on the shoulders. A close grip bench press primarily works the triceps and the front delts.

Chest Exercises

Exercise 23   Dumbbell Flye

BASIC EXERCISE Where a press uses two joints, a flye uses one. Too often, I see flyes and presses in-breeding—creating a weird, hybrid "press-flye" that isn't too effective because the origin of motion isn't clear. A press is a push. A flye is a round embrace.

Movement Always start by holding the weights together, up in the air (to avoid overstretching the shoulders on your first motion). Elbows are "soft" but fixed—they shouldn't bend or straighten during the exercise. As your arms open to the side, lift your sternum to the ceiling. Be careful not to drop the weights too low or arch the back. As you bring your arms together, raise your chest *even more.* Add an extra "squeeze" in the chest at the top of the lift.

Drawing with the weight Your hands start at 12 o'clock. Lower to 3 and 9 o'clock position. Your elbows can be a little lower. Return to 12 o'clock. Be sure to draw good round arcs.

Safety tips Control the weights on the way down and avoid bouncing your shoulders. Also, be sure to keep weights on the vertical line of gravity. On an incline, the angle can be disorienting, and thus it's easy to lift the weights forward or back. Be sure you lift straight up and down.

Targeted muscles Chest and front shoulder.

Function A lot of simple daily tasks incorporate this motion—from cleaning windows to washing the car. It's also used in tennis and swimming.

Aesthetics Where a press puts on strength, meat and power, a flye etches in fine points—cleavage, the sexy tie-ins between the arm, shoulder and chest.

Tricks of the trade Keep your shoulders back—it's easy to forget.

No cheating Try not to bang the dumbbells together at the top—and thus risk losing "the squeeze" in the chest. Keep constant tension in the muscles.

Visualization Imagine you're hugging a very large person.

Variation Try this same exercise using a bench and two floor cables. Also, try lifting just halfway—i.e., to 10 and 2 o'clock (and hold it there for a moment). This puts more constant stress on the chest—and less of a shift into the shoulder joint. You can also do flyes with cables, lying on a flat, decline or incline bench. Try crossing the handles at the wrist, since cables, unlike dumbbells, supply resistance in this part of the motion.

REMINDERS:

1. Lift from shoulder, not elbow

2. *Lift* chest as arms come together

3. Beware of dropping weights too low

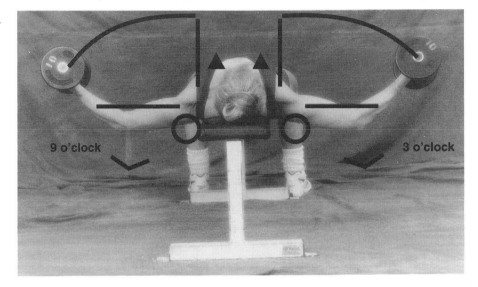

9 o'clock

3 o'clock

Chest Exercises

Exercise 24 Standing Cable Crossovers (or Cable Flyes)

INTERMEDIATE EXERCISE Although the motion here is similar to that of the dumbbell flye, this exercise is more challenging because it's done standing—thus, the torso must be stable.

Movement Stand in the center and slightly in front of two "cross cables." If you need extra stability, put one foot forward. Your torso can be vertical or slightly inclined forward from 10 to 45 degrees. Both the angle of your spine and your body in relation to the cables are variable—yet the posture stays the same.

Drawing with the weight Once again, your hands start at 3 and 9 o'clock and end either at 12 o'clock, or cross at the midline to 1 and 11 o'clock. When crossing, be sure to alternate which hand goes on top.

Safety tip Be sure not to let the cables or band get away from you. Avoid jerking your arms behind your shoulders.

Targeted muscles Chest and front shoulder.

Function Same as regular flyes.

Aesthetics More cleavage, more fingers of definition etched horizontally across the chest.

Tricks of the trade To get a better feel for this, do one arm at a time. Spot the opposite hand on the working shoulder, to keep it down and back.

No cheating No rounding of the torso, no windup move to hurl the weight with momentum.

Visualization There's something very satisfying about this move—and it's a great way to finish off a chest workout. Presses build the cake. Flyes and crossovers put on the icing.

Variation Try this from floor cables, instead of overheads. Just make sure that your weight stacks are light enough. Coming from the floor is much more challenging on the front delts. If you don't have access to cables, you can use some form of elastic resistance. You'll need to anchor one end of the band at your side, slightly above and behind your shoulders. Tie tubing or a band around a pole or put the Lifeline Gym loop attachment through a door jam and close the door. Position your body as you would if you were using cables, slightly in front of the pulleys. With elastic resistance, however, it's best to do one arm at a time because that fixed point will only serve one side of your pectorals. You could tie the ends of two bands between two poles and stand in the center, but two such poles are hard to find. Tying and looping bands always makes me nervous. There's no guarantee that they won't come undone, snap you in the face or break. So, be warned and be careful.

Chest Exercises

REMINDERS:

1. Keep torso steady
2. *Lift* chest as arms come together

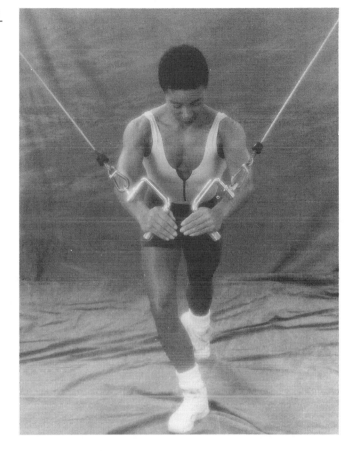

Shoulder Exercises

Exercise 25   Lateral Raises

BASIC EXERCISE

The shoulder joint is delicate and easily injured. This particular exercise is a one-joint move and thus hangs lots of weight off that shoulder. Common errors include:

- using too heavy weight—even with bent elbows
- using too much lower back motion and momentum
- banging weights at the bottom, to "wind up" for the next rep
- lifting arms too high, thus impinging the joint and transferring the work-load into the trapezius (upper back).

The following variations are more gentle and strict and simultaneously work and preserve the shoulders.

Movement

With dumbbells. Try this one seated on a bench to minimize the temptation to swing the torso (although you can do the same thing standing, letting the dumbbells down in front of your body). Keep your elbows soft—not locked—wrists straight, shoulders down. Raise your arms parallel to the floor—or an inch higher but no more. Lift your arms from 6 o'clock to 3 and 9 o'clock. *Lying on side incline with dumbbell.* This one minimizes the "dead zone" found at the bottom of the motion in a regular lateral raise (and thus incorporates more muscle fibers). Set the bench to a 45-degree angle. Lie on your side,

REMINDERS:

1. Keep elbows soft, shoulders down

2. Avoid raising arms too high (this impinges shoulder joint)

3. Keep torso still

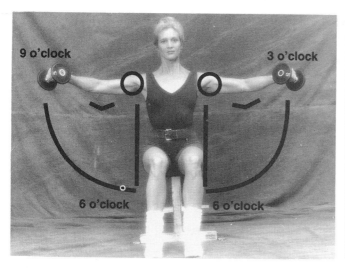

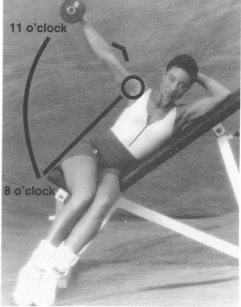

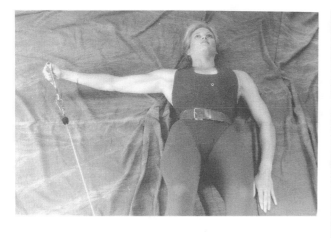

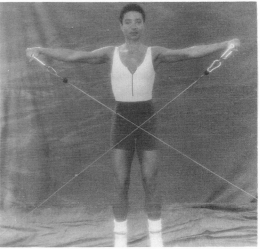

resting your head on an arm or a rolled up towel. Start at 8 o'clock, raise to 11 o'clock. (It's the same r.o.m. tilted sideways.)

Lying on floor, with one floor cable. Lie on your back, with your arm at your side, holding a single cable. Again, lift from 6 to 9 o'clock. A good way to avoid the "dead zone," it's also very safe for the back.

Standing cable. Stand in the center of a cable crossover, holding floor handles crossed in front of your hips. Again raise from 6 o'clock to 9 and 3.

Safety tips	In standing exercises, be extra careful to keep your back still. Avoid lifting your arms too high, especially when you can't see them in all exercises. Also avoid pointing your thumbs down as if you're pouring out water—another compromise to rotators and shoulder joint stability.
Targeted muscles	Front and middle deltoid.
Main moving joint	Shoulder. A lateral raise is basically a "flye" for shoulders.
Function	Shoulders assist in all upper body motions. Since shoulders are so prone to injury, perhaps even more so than backs and knees, it's crucial that they're strong enough to meet demands—and worked intelligently. Badly trained shoulders eventually end up injured.
Aesthetics	Shoulders define the line of the upper body. A well-toned shoulder adds shape to arms and lends an air of power to the physique (one reason shoulder pads are popular).
Tricks of the trade	Every time you raise an arm, pull the shoulder *down.*
No cheating	Avoid going fast with heavy weight just to complete the reps. Slow down. Squeeze. Join the Save the Shoulder Foundation.
Visualization	Be like a slow bird flapping its wings.
Variation	For seated raises, try angling your torso forward about 5 to 10 degrees to minimize any wobble in the back.

Shoulder Exercises

Exercise 26   Shoulder Presses

BASIC EXERCISE

Although this is a basic exercise, you should beware any time you raise a weight overhead because it's tempting to arch the back. Also, presses with a bar behind the head put too much external rotation on the shoulder joint. If you must do presses with a bar, bring the bar to your *collarbone*, rather than behind the head. Dumbbells don't cause that problem of excessive rotation and allow you to work each side independently—thus giving the weaker side an equal chance. There are two variations on the dumbbell presses—the standard and the strict or "box" presses.

Movement

Regardless of the version, each press should initiate from a spot where your thumbs would point at your neck if you weren't holding weights. If you hold them too high you'll have a shortened r.o.m.; too low causes your shoulders to drop, which could lead to pain in the joint.

Standard presses. The weights touch overhead. You'll be able to use more weight on this version, simply because the work is shared by deltoids and trapezius—so you've got two muscle groups in the act. Draw an A shape with the weights coming together in a point overhead.

Strict or "box" presses. Keep your arms parallel throughout the motion—don't bring the weights together. You'll need lighter weight than above since this move focuses more on deltoids. Keep the weights directly over your shoulders.

Drawing with the weight

As you lower the weights, keep your arms perpendicular to the floor. Draw clean parallel or intersecting lines as you press.

Safety tips

Avoid locking your elbows. If your shoulders bother you, try rotating your thumbs so they point behind you, about 45 degrees to 90 degrees. Also, beware that the further out your hands are from the shoulder joint, the riskier it is on the tendon. Be sure that weights press straight up on the line of gravity, not up and forward. Once you feel your back begin to arch, finish the set with lighter weight.

Targeted muscles

Front and middle deltoid.

Main moving joints

Shoulder and elbow.

Function

Not many of us do this motion in life or even in sports. We do this whenever we have occasion to press a box onto a high shelf.

Aesthetics

This exercise adds shoulder shape and size.

Left: *Standard press.*
Right: *Box press.*

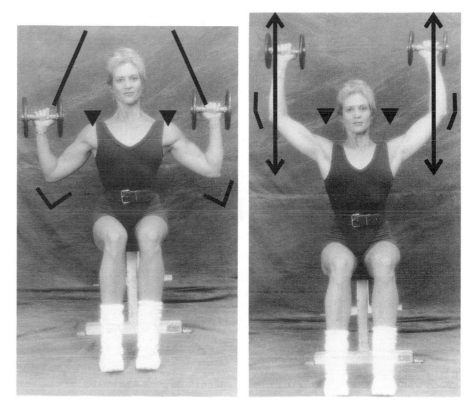

Tricks of the trade	As you press up, think "down" with your shoulders. No shrugging.
No cheating	Beware of arching your back to complete the reps.
Visualization	Imagine the weights travel up and down on tracks. Also, pretend you're a robot with only one moving part—the arms. Program your torso to keep still.
Variation	When you fail with both arms, try alternating one at a time. When you do this one in a machine, try facing *into* the bench, to position the handles in front of your shoulders—both for variety's sake and to ease any pain caused by rotation.

Shoulder Exercises

Exercise 27   Front Cable Raise

BASIC EXERCISE   Normally I don't recommend front raises, not with dumbbells, anyway. These work the front portion of the shoulder muscle, which gets enough work with chest exercises. It's wiser, therefore, to focus on the middle and rear parts of the shoulder. However, this particular version of a front raise greatly fatigues the *medial* as well as the front delt, causing an enormous pump—without compromising the spine.

Movement   Lie on the floor, with a rolling EZ curl bar (bent bar) attached to a floor cable. Bend your knees slightly (with fully bent knees you won't have sufficient r.o.m. for the bar). Rest the bar on your thighs. Take an overhand grip on the bar, about shoulder distance apart. Press your shoulders down and back and "puff up" your chest before you lift.

Drawing with the weight   Start the motion at 3 o'clock and lift the bar to 12 o'clock, no higher—or it's off into the "dead zone."

Safety tips   Use slow, steady motion, lifting and lowering. Avoid jerking the weight or banging plates—it's jarring for shoulder joint.

Targeted muscles   Front and middle portion of shoulder.

Main moving joint   Shoulder only. This is yet another flye. Keep elbows soft but fixed.

Function   Front delts assist in all pushing motions. Middle delts help lift your arms out to the side. Both assist in many sports—swimming, dancing, tennis, volleyball—not to mention raising a fork to your mouth!

Aesthetics   This exercise is particularly valuable for etching in the "point" of the middle deltoid, between your biceps and triceps, adding a sleek, elegant look to the arm.

Tricks of the trade   Try working the negatives very slowly. And be humble when it comes to choosing an appropriate weight. On a "light" weight stack, beginners average 5 to 10 lbs. Also, press your heels into the ground for extra abdominal support.

No cheating   No lifting up beyond 12 o'clock.

Visualization   This motion is like a two-handed salute.

Variation   Try doing this with a single handle.

Shoulder Exercises

1. Keep elbows soft
2. Press heels into floor for extra abdominal support

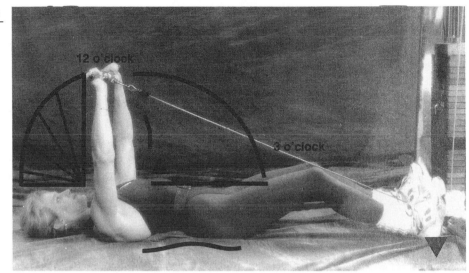

Shoulder Exercises

Exercise 28   Half Upright Rows

BASIC EXERCISE   Traditional upright rows target the shoulders and the trapezius—with a wide grip emphasizing shoulders, a narrow grip the trapezius. People who feel pain in their rotators in traditional uprights might benefit from this variation.

Movement   Set a floor cable as for the last exercise. In fact, this makes a great "super-set" with cable front raises. Do this immediately after the cable front raises, taking no more than a 15-second rest between the two sets. Pull the bar to your sternum (just below the breasts).

Drawing with the weight   Keep the bar floating just above your torso, pulling in a clean horizontal line, parallel to the floor.

Safety tips   With your back supported on the floor, this is a safe position and safe exercise for the shoulders. Be sure, however, to use slow, controlled motion on the way up and down.

Targeted muscles   Shoulders.

Main moving joints   Shoulders and elbows—keep your wrists straight.

Function   Any time you pick up a suitcase, you do a modified version of this motion.

Aesthetics   Like the front raise, this exercise allows you to create new shape and definition without taxing the shoulder joint. It also doesn't build up the trapezius (or "traps"), one muscle that looks unattractive on a woman when it's too well developed. (For this reason, I don't recommend shrugs with heavy weight. Thick traps tighten already tight neck muscles and give shoulders the look of a linebacker's.)

Tricks of the trade   Before lifting the bar, press your shoulders *out* to initiate the move. Keep your chest lifting throughout.

No cheating   Don't pull the bar too high or let your elbows rest on floor. Work slowly to keep constant tension in your shoulders.

Visualization   Imagine you're raising up the front of your skirt.

Variation   Try a single handle.

Shoulder Exercises

REMINDERS:

1. Keep bar approximately 1 inch over body

2. Don't let elbows rest on floor

3. Press shoulders down and chest up as you lift

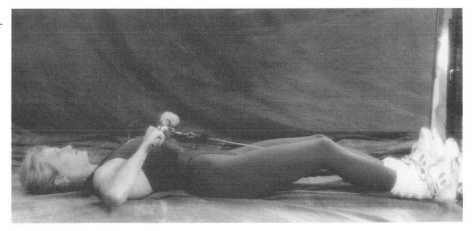

Shoulder Exercises

Exercise 29   Rear Delt Variations

BASIC EXERCISE

If your body was a map of the United States, the rear delts would be Rhode Island. This portion of the body is small and tucked between two larger muscles. But it serves an important function—rear delts are "good posture" muscles. They get some involvement with shoulder and back exercises but they also need their own, undiluted attention—and because they're so small, they can only handle modest weight.

Movement

Rear delt motions are all flyes, one-joint moves only. Don't bend your elbows to lift more weight. Be humble and benefit more.

Lying on side, dumbbell raise. This is my favorite because it looks so innocent, yet does the job so well. Lie sideways on a bench. (You might get better balance if you support your head on the bottom hand and extend the top leg for counterweight.) Keep your working arm directly in front of the shoulder joint.

Drawing with the weight

Begin the motion at 8 o'clock; raise it up to 10 o'clock. If you raise much higher, the rear delt will cease working.

Lying on back using cables

Set up a bench between two cross cables. Grab the top cables with the opposite hands and lie on your back on the bench.

Drawing with the weight

Start with cables crossed, hands together at 12 o'clock. Open your arms to 9 and 3 o'clock. This is the reverse of a chest cable flye.

Safety tips

Be sure not to jerk the arm too far behind the torso and avoid adding elbow. When you fail, continue with less weight or resistance—or even no weight at all. The weight of the arm on the side-lying version can be surprisingly heavy—a good way to add reps at the end of a set.

Targeted muscles

Rear delts.

Main moving joint

Shoulder.

Function

Strong rear delts prevent slouching.

Aesthetics

Chiseled rear delts add the look of a finishing touch—the mark of someone who's been at this for a while.

Tricks of the trade

On the dumbbell exercise, rotate your arm slightly so the thumb points to the floor for a more finely tuned isolation.

No cheating

No bending the elbows or twisting the torso!

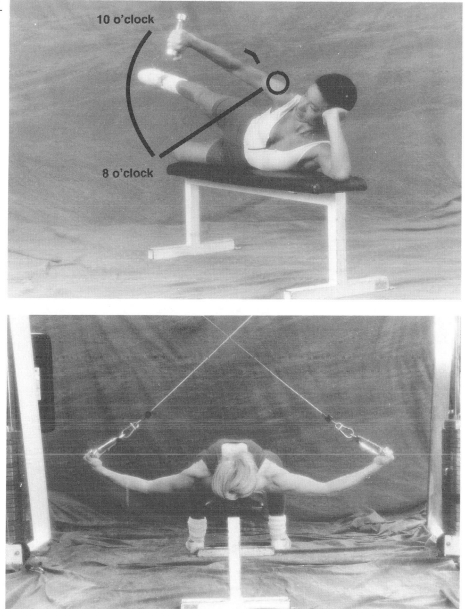

Visualization See the tiny triangular shapes of the rear delts in your mind's eye. Let them light up with every rep.

Variation Try the reverse cable flyes standing up—as if doing a backwards cable crossover.

Shoulder Exercises

Exercise 30   External & Internal Rotators

BASIC & REHAB EXERCISE   The rotator cuff in the shoulder is actually made up of four small muscles. External rotators get injured more frequently—especially during military presses or pull-downs behind the neck and in heavy bench presses. These two exercises are preventives and can also be part of a rehab program for already injured or vulnerable rotators.

Movement   *External rotation with dumbbell.* Lie sideways on a flat bench. Hold a light dumbbell in the top hand and position the top elbow into your hip, so it's stable.

Drawing with the weight   Rotate your forearm from 8 to 11 o'clock.
Internal rotation with dumbbell. In the same position, put the weight in the lower hand.

Drawing with the weight   Lift from 8 or 9 to 12 o'clock, depending on your flexibility.

Safety tip   Avoid trying to achieve more r.o.m. here, especially if it hurts.

Targeted muscles   Shoulder rotators.

Main moving joint   Elbow only!

Function   These muscles assist in the majority of arm motions—and are especially important for swimming freestyle and performing the tennis serve.

Aesthetics   The outward benefits of this are invisible.

Tricks of the trade   Use minimal weight and resistance. Weight that's too heavy could cause further damage. Also, fatigue comes on quickly.

No cheating   Be sure not to use the shoulder joint.

Visualization   Imagine you're a robot with only one moving hinge on your body.

Variation   If you have a resistance band, hold it with *both* hands, with your elbows braced on your hips (as if pointing two loaded "six-guns"). Pull band apart with both hands, starting at 12 o'clock, opening to 10 and 2.

Shoulder Exercises

REMINDER:

1. These are small, delicate muscles; use light weight

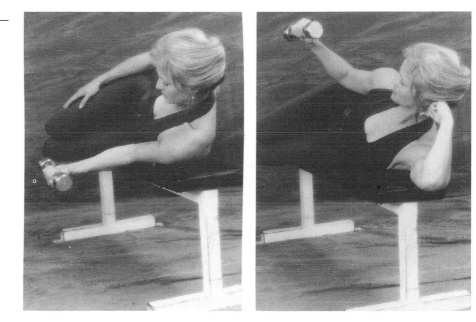

Biceps Exercises

Exercise 31   Barbell Curl

BASIC EXERCISE   The pure curl is simplicity at its best. It's not fancy and it always works.

Movement   *With a straight bar.* As you know, this is a simple one-joint move. Many people add all sorts of variations—EZ curl bars, bars with rotating handles, an "arm blaster" to hold the elbows in place—all of which "address" muscles at different angles. But to do the unadulterated standing curl, simply grab a barbell and hang your arms close by your sides.

Drawing with the weight   Raise the bar from 6 to 10 o'clock. Squeeze your muscles at the top and lower with control.

Safety tips   Keep your lower back still, shoulders down and back. Be careful not to rest your elbows on your hips or collapse the chest.

Targeted muscles   Biceps.

Main moving joint   Elbow.

Function   Biceps assist in all pulling motions—such as lifting a suitcase, swimming freestyle, rowing.

Aesthetics   Tell someone you're lifting weights and the first thing they'll want to see is your biceps. Biceps size still represents a prize for the weight lifter's ego.

Tricks of the trade   Press upper arm into torso (as if holding a pencil under each armpit), for more control over the motion and an impressive pump in the biceps.

No cheating   Don't just lower halfway down. That's cheating! Lower *all* the way.

Visualization   Imagine that your elbows are bolted to your hips. Keep them down!

Variations   A wide grip doesn't involve both biceps and brachialis muscles to the same extent as a narrow grip. A wide grip mostly stresses the top (medial) or bulbous part of the biceps. A narrow grip also uses the deeper brachialis (a muscle that helps give biceps size). Vary the grip size at your whim, but be aware that a narrow grip gives greater, more visible benefits.

Biceps Exercises

REMINDERS:

1. Keep shoulders down and back
2. Keep torso steady

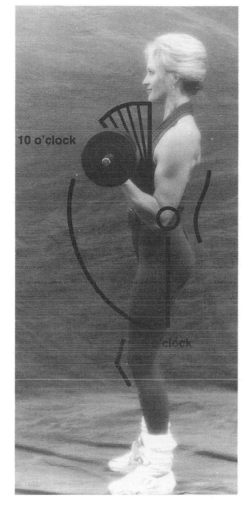

10 o'clock

o'clock

Biceps Exercises

Exercise 32   Dumbbell Curl

BASIC EXERCISE

Although logic dictates that if you can curl a 30 lb. barbell, you should be able to curl 15 lb. dumbbells, this isn't always the case. You may have to drop down to 10 lb. dumbbells to accommodate a weaker side and/or maintain form.

Movement

The range of motion is nearly the same for dumbbells. However, the hand position you choose can determine which biceps muscles you work the most. To take the most advantage of the biceps' ability to rotate as well as lift the arm, start the move with your palms facing your sides. As you raise the dumbbells rotate your palms up. (Maintaining a palm-in grip throughout—otherwise called a hammer curl—focuses more on just the lateral head—which lives under the more obvious medial head. This is also easier to do.)

Drawing with the weight

Lift from 6 to 2 o'clock.

Safety tips

Be cautious not to overtwist your elbows when adding rotation.

Main moving joints

Elbows. Wrists are involved when rotating the palms outward, but don't "break" them.

Function

Again, this motion assists in all pulling moves and, in particular, helps work arms one at a time—to even out your strength.

Aesthetics

Women may say, "I don't want bulging biceps" and thus stay away from biceps exercises in general. But biceps, when strengthened, help bring out the very beautiful line of definition shared by your shoulders and triceps.

Tricks of the trade

Try doing this one arm at a time for better focus and more intensity, rather than two at a time or alternating.

No cheating

Don't just crank out reps. Do each rep mindfully and squeeze your biceps at the top.

Visualization

Arm muscles respond well when you add an extra "squeeze" with each contraction. At the top of each lift, imagine you're wringing water from a towel.

Variation

Try "running the rack." Do 4 to 6 reps with heavy weight, then immediately do 4 to 6 more with moderate weight, then finish off with 4 to 6 light-weight reps. Whew!

Biceps Exercises

REMINDERS:

1. Keep shoulders down and back
2. Add an extra "squeeze" at the top of each contraction.
3. Keep torso still

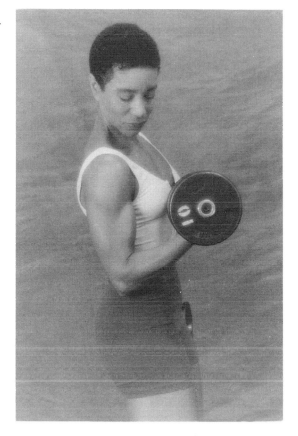

Biceps Exercises

Exercise 33   Incline Cable Curl

INTERMEDIATE EXERCISE

The only thing that separates this from a basic exercise is the inclined torso and greater r.o.m. If you're comfortable in this position, go ahead and make it a basic. This exercise works my biceps better than any other—and helped my arms grow from puny to respectable. In this position you get more stress at the bottom portion of the lift and the cable lets you feel more constant resistance—without "dead zones."

Movement

Set up a floor cable and single handle. Standing, face away from the pulley. Put one leg forward to stabilize your torso. Keep your elbow down at your side and your arm in line with your spine as you curl.

Drawing with the weight

This time, curl from 7 to 2 o'clock.

Safety tips

If you're very flexible, be wary of hyperextending your elbows in the stretch position, stressing the elbow tendon. Also avoid all swinging from the shoulder.

Targeted muscles

Biceps.

Main moving joint

Elbow.

Function

Assists all pulling moves.

Aesthetics

Since biceps muscles don't have much fat on them (fat is stored in the triceps), a little work can begin to show up quickly. But don't worry about getting "big arms."

Tricks of the trade

Don't let your upper arm move at all.

No cheating

Beware of curling too high, swinging the shoulder and elbow, or bending the wrist.

Visualization

Imagine the biceps is a small balloon, inserted into your arm and each rep blows in more air: Feel it expand. Also, imagine your upper arm is bolted to your rib cage.

Variation

If you have a rotating handle, try this palm in, rotating your forearm to palm out at the top of the lift, for a fuller contraction.

Biceps Exercises

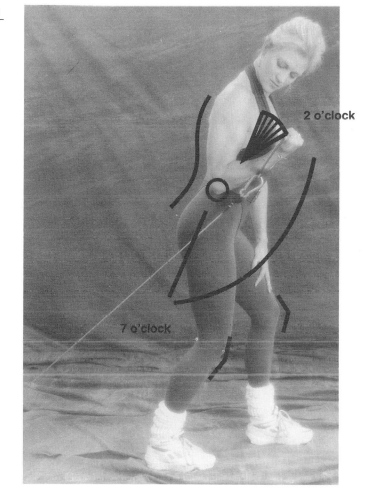

2 o'clock

7 o'clock

Biceps Exercises

Exercise 34   Preacher Curls

INTERMEDIATE EXERCISE

Preachers are called preachers because the bench puts you in a position for prayer—which seems appropriate in the final reps. This isn't an important exercise for beginners—its pluses are more esoteric. This exercise puts "the peak" on the biceps or the icing on the cake. But why worry about icing, if you haven't yet built the cake?

The main problem with preachers is that bench. You have to position yourself just right—not too high, not too low—your armpits on the curve of the bench, your back in neutral (the tendency is to round both shoulders forward). Most people get more control if they do one arm at a time and sit in a three-quarters front position. This keeps the shoulders from rolling forward and stealing all the action—and lets you spot yourself when you fail. This elbows-forward position puts most of the mechanical stress on the lower part of the motion—thus it's a good one for people with "short" biceps because, to some extent, it helps fill in the "gaps." However, this is also genetic. Length of muscle belly can't be altered much.

Movement

Begin the motion at 8 o'clock and lift to 12 o'clock or just shy of it—but not higher or you're in the dead zone. At the top of the lift, squeeze your biceps, then lower all the way.

Safety tips

Be careful not to hyperextend your elbows as you straighten your arm. Keep your shoulders back, down and motionless. When you hit the "sticking point," spot yourself gently—or, if you must use a bar, get assistance from a spotter.

Targeted muscles

Biceps.

Main moving joint

Elbow.

Function

All pulling, lifting motions—plus rowing and racquet sports.

Aesthetics

You may not want big biceps when you start lifting, but after a while, your tastes may change. You may then hit up against the frustrating truth—that for most of us, it takes time to grow impressive arms.

Tricks of the trade

Try adding a slight rotation of the wrist (with your pinkie toward your shoulder) to etch in the "outer" head of the biceps.

REMINDERS:

1. Sitting sideways keeps shoulder back
2. Avoid hyperextending elbows

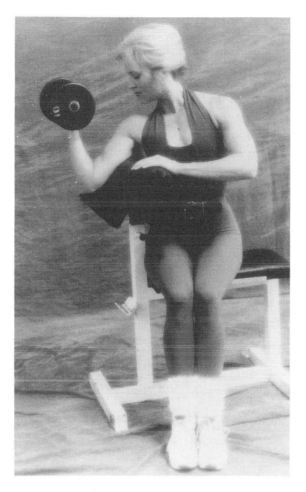

No cheating	Don't shorten your range of motion at the bottom and extend it at the top. Keep it honest.
Visualization	Imagine your arm is a big nutcracker and your biceps a giant walnut. With every rep, crack the nut!
Variation	Try this with a cable and single handle.

Triceps Exercises

Exercise 35   Press-Downs

BASIC EXERCISE   The size of the triceps determines the shape and size of the arm. It's also where much body fat gets stored—like the upper body's version of a thigh. The r.o.m. for triceps is the same as for the biceps, in reverse.

Movement   Stand in front of a rotating cable bar—bent, angled or straight—attached to an overhead cable. (A bar that rotates is much easier on your hands.) A narrow grip of 4 to 6 inches wide involves more triceps "heads," but you can change this for variety. Keep your shoulders back and don't let your posture "cave in" as you press the bar down. As with biceps work, don't raise your elbows forward, and remember to keep your wrists straight.

Drawing with the weight   Start the motion at 10 o'clock. Bring the bar down to your thighs, to between 7 and 6 o'clock. If you want more r.o.m., step further away from the cable and slightly incline your torso. Also try this with a single handle and a palm-up grip. Some handles let you rotate the palm into the body at the bottom of the move—for a final, delicious squeeze.

Safety tips   Don't let your elbows lift or your shoulders move. This transfers work out of the triceps! Beware of getting a momentum-boosted "windup" with every rep.

Targeted muscles   Triceps—especially long and lateral heads.

Main moving joint   Elbows.

Function   This exercise assists with all pressing motions used in sports and everyday life.

Aesthetics   Your overall arm "tone" largely depends on the strength and definition of your triceps.

Tricks of the trade   As with biceps, give triceps an extra "squeeze" when muscles are contracted.

No cheating   Get your shoulders back, keep your elbows by your hips. Don't bang the plates.

Visualization   Again imagine your upper arms are bolted to your sides. The elbow is the only moving joint.

Variation   Try doing the EZ curl bar with a palm-up grip—it's much harder. Also, try this with a rope handle. Press down and then extend your arms out in an A shape, to bring in the medial head of the triceps.

Triceps Exercises

REMINDERS:

1. Keep elbows close to sides

2. Add extra "squeeze" when muscles are contracted.

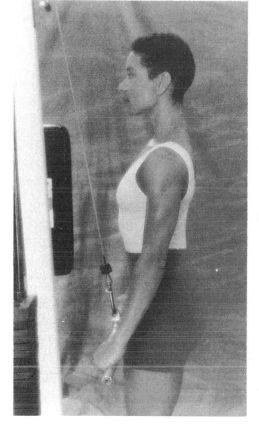

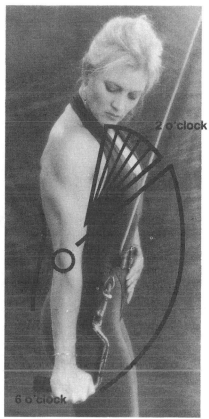

Triceps Exercises

Exercise 36   Dumbbell Triceps Extension

BASIC EXERCISE This exercise helps firm up "the jiggle"—those silky, perfumed "batwings" that flap off the upper arms of grandmothers.

Movement Sit or stand, holding the weight overhead, with your working arm straight up. Lower the weight below your opposite ear (so that if you didn't have the weight in hand, you'd be able to touch the thumb to the outside of your neck). Make sure the elbow stays pointed up to the ceiling the whole time—if it points to the wall you're no longer working the triceps, or much of anything. Keep your shoulders down and stable.

Drawing with the weight Start the movement at 12 o'clock, then lower to 4 o'clock.

Safety tips Any time you take a weight overhead, pay extra attention to keeping a neutral spine. Also, to spot yourself, hold the elbow of your working arm stationary. (Just make sure you put your spotting arm *in front* of your face, not behind your head, or you'll get in your own way!) In this position, you're ready to grab the dumbbell if you fail. Also be careful not to drop the weight too low, as this could "hang" too much weight off the elbow tendon.

Targeted muscles All three heads of the triceps: a good investment of time and energy.

Main moving joint Elbow.

Function Triceps assist in all pushing motions. Especially useful for a tennis serve, volleyball, swimming the breaststroke or even just pushing a box onto a shelf.

Aesthetics The triceps make up a bigger portion of the arm than the biceps. Thus, it's the muscle that adds the most size, shape and definition to the arm.

Tricks of the trade Keep your wrists straight for the maximum load on the triceps.

No cheating Go for the complete r.o.m.

Visualization Picture scrubbing your back with a back brush . . .

Variation Try using a floor cable for this. Also play with half-reps in the lower portion of the movement—going from 4 to 2 o'clock—a torch song to the triceps.

REMINDERS:

1. Keep upper arm stationary and wrists straight

2. Keep working shoulder down

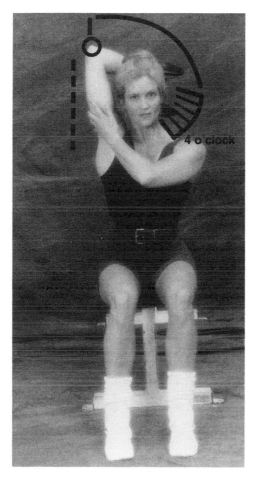

4 o'clock

Triceps Exercises

Exercise 37   French Press

INTERMEDIATE EXERCISE

Why this is called a French press, I don't know. I've also heard it called "Suicide," which is a better description but doesn't exactly inspire confidence. Yes, this exercise takes some control and initial strength to do well. Otherwise, you can bonk yourself in the forehead. So be careful. Once you have a foundation of triceps strength, this is an excellent way to work all three heads of the triceps at once.

Movement

Work on a flat bench or a slight decline. Lying on your back, angle your upper arms about 10 degrees above your head. This position, especially on the decline, puts constant stress on the triceps and keeps it a one-joint move. Bringing your arms straight up can add the shoulder and put you in the "dead zone." Keep your arms parallel throughout.

Drawing with the weight

Lower the bar from 1 to 4 o'clock. Make sure the bar goes towards the *top* of your head when you lower—don't aim for your eyebrows!

Safety tips

If you're unsure of this, have a spotter on hand. Lower slowly.

Targeted muscles

All three heads of the triceps.

Main moving joint

Elbow.

Function

All pushing motions.

Aesthetics

A ripply, seductive, sinewy muscle dancing around under healthy skin!

Tricks of the trade

If you use an EZ curl bar (an angled barbell) the thumbs rotate up. This slight rotation also rotates and stabilizes the shoulder. This position makes it easier to keep your upper arm still.

No cheating

Keep your wrists straight. If you can do this confidently, a thumbless grip helps keep the wrists "in line."

Visualization

Imagine that your arms move on parallel grooves, as if set on railroad tracks. Don't let them deviate.

Variation

Finish this motion with a super-set of bench presses with the same narrow grip you used for the French press.

Triceps Exercises

REMINDERS:

1. Angle straight arm to 1 o'clock to avoid "dead zone"

2. Keep arms parallel, don't open elbows

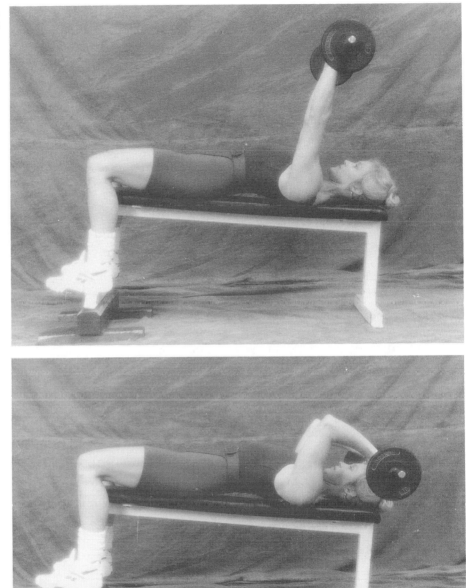

Triceps Exercises

Exercise 38   Triceps Kickback

BASIC EXERCISE   Probably the most widely performed triceps exercise, it's most effective when done with subtlety.

Movement   Support one knee and the same side arm on a bench, bending forward so your spine is either parallel to floor or at least on a 45-degree angle. The working elbow (away from the bench) should be slightly behind the back. Holding a dumbbell, gently extend your arm to straight.

Drawing with the weight   Start the motion at 6 o'clock and straighten your arm to 3 o'clock. It's not necessary to bring your hand back to 7 o'clock when you're holding a dumbbell. That takes you off the vertical gravity line and puts you in a "dead zone."

Safety tips   Beware of using so much weight or resistance that your shoulder rolls forward—irritating the biceps tendon and overinvolving the front head of the shoulder, also not permitting you to fully extend your arm.

Targeted muscles   Triceps—particularly the lateral and medial heads—which adds shape and size respectively to the triceps.

Main moving joint   Elbow.

Function   Again, all pushing motions.

Aesthetics   This exercise helps chisel in the horseshoe-shaped triceps.

Tricks of the trade   Pressing the upper arm into your torso (as if gripping a $100 bill under each armpit) helps stabilize the shoulder, thus preventing a "pinched" feeling in the biceps tendon.

No cheating   No hurling the weight or whacking away at the poor elbow. And beware of using extra heavy weight and a shortened r.o.m. In such a small muscle, the squeeze is king!

Visualization   Imagine you have a cape draped over your shoulders. To keep the cape from falling forward, hold your shoulders back and down. Don't round forward, or the cape will fall over you.

Variations   Try varying your grip—palms down, up or in (when your arm is extended) to see which one gives you the most control. Palms down is hardest. Also, try this with a floor cable or resistance band, anchored under supporting hand or tied to a fixed pole. This allows you to use resistance from 7 o'clock to 3 o'clock.

Triceps Exercises

REMINDERS:

1. Keep elbow close to your side
2. Pull shoulder back and down

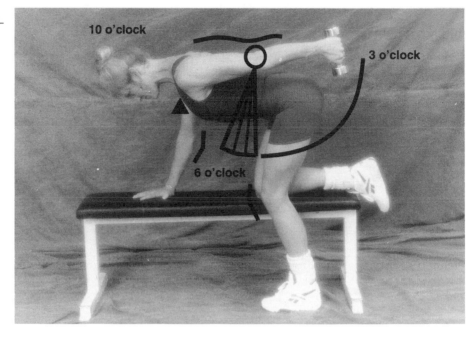

10 o'clock

3 o'clock

6 o'clock

Abdominal Exercises

Exercise 39   Reverse Curls

BASIC EXERCISE   It's hard to be "centered" without a strong center. The abdominals mark the intersection between the lower and upper body and are essential to all moves that require stabilizing one half of the body while the other half exerts—as in a golf swing, a tennis stroke, karate kick, throwing a Frisbee, lifting a box, etc. Strong "abs" insure better body placement, minimize the risk of lower back problems and also act as a girdle for internal organs.

But too often, people confuse abdominal work with rounding the back. Thus, some people who boast about doing 500 crunches actually have mushy abs because they're only relying on the rounding motion, momentum and using hip flexors—not squeezing the intended muscles (the rectus abdominus and obliques).

Other common errors include:

- Full sit-ups. After the shoulders lift off the floor, the work transfers into the back and hip flexors, rendering the majority of the move useless and risky.

- Double leg raises, especially with straight legs. These primarily use hip flexors; abs work only as a stabilizer. This motion can put the lower back at high risk.

The following exercises are basic and usable for all levels. If you do them slowly and hold the contractions—adding a little pulse here and there for variety—you won't need 500 or even 50 reps. You should be glad to get to 10!

Movement   Lie on your back, with your knees over your hips, so that the back is slightly pelvic tilted. For more stability, hold onto the top of a bench or, if you're on the floor, an overhead pole. (With nothing to hold onto, rest your hands by your hips.) Before you move anything, contract your abdominals (as if someone just punched you in the stomach). *Then* curl your tailbone up towards your belly button, lifting the pelvis off the floor. As you lower, fight against gravity. Use the negatives.

Drawing with the weight   Lift your tailbone from 9 o'clock to 10 o'clock. Slowly lower your hips, keeping tension on the abdominal muscles even on negatives. Count it like this: "Contract 1-2, lift 3-4, squeeze 5-6, lower 7-8."

Safety tip   Beware of being overly ambitious and curling your whole spine off the floor: Unless you've got the strength to control it, you might find yourself in an

REMINDERS:

1. Contract
abdominals
before you lift

2. Lower tailbone
slowly

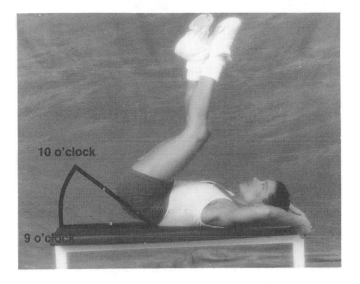

unsafe back stretch without any abdominal contraction at all. If you experience neck or shoulder tension, try rolling up a sweatshirt or a towel and placing it under your neck. Beware of putting a "death grip" on the bench or the pole.

Targeted muscles	Rectus abdominus—i.e., the belly.
Main moving joints	The vertebrae in the lower back—not the hips!
Function	We use abdominals in all motions, plus breathing, sitting, standing, singing, talking, laughing.
Aesthetics	Strong, cut, washboard abs are the result of strengthening, aerobics and a steady life of low-fat eating. It's possible to be strong but still have muscles hidden under fat. Also, the "flat tummy" for some is an impossible dream. No matter how hard we work or how lean we become, many of us still have bellies that are naturally rounded (and quite sexy). Sometimes it's important to let these bellies "hang loose" so we can breathe fully, let air down there, sing with power, move from the center. A strong center, therefore, isn't just about tight muscles, but muscles that can be both tight and loose, adapting to different demands.
Tricks of the trade	Try holding your tailbone off the floor and gently pulse upwards.
No cheating	Don't hurl yourself up. You might strain the lower back.
Visualization	Imagine that your abs are wet sponges. With every rep, squeeze out all the water.
Variation	Do this with your knees tucked towards one shoulder at a time—to bring in the obliques.

Abdominal Exercises

Exercise 40   Rollbacks

INTERMEDIATE EXERCISE

The secret of this exercise isn't the lift but the lower. Thus, all the action takes place in the negative. The other secret is to lower only partway down the decline bench.

Movement

Curl your feet under the pads of the decline bench (if you have a flat bench, bend your knees and secure your feet). Lower the torso no more than halfway down the bench, hold for a moment and lift.

Drawing with the weight

Start with your head at the 1 o'clock position, then slowly lower to 2—or for very advanced people, 3 o'clock—taking about 4–5 seconds to get there. Lift back to 1 o'clock. For extra support, hold on to the bench or your knees.

Safety tips

By no means should you go down to the point where your lower back hurts.

Targeted muscles

Rectus abdominus. Also, because the abdominals work to stabilize the torso, this works deep down into the transverse abdominus (the deepest abdominal muscles, which act as a girdle for our internal organs).

Main moving joints

Vertebrae in lower and middle back.

Function

This strengthens abdominal muscles deep down towards the pubic bone.

Aesthetics

This helps chisel in the "six-pack" chunks of muscle visible in "washboard abs."

Tricks of the trade

It's too stressful even for very strong people to rest their heads in their hands (the weight of the arms makes the torso too heavy). Keep your arms by your side—or cross them over your chest. Think of curling and uncurling your spine, rather than lowering a stiff, straight torso.

No cheating

Don't lower too low (using hip flexors) or come up too high (into the dead zone).

Visualization

As you curl and uncurl, do so from the navel. Like the Pillsbury Dough Boy, "marshmallow" around a giant finger. Let the shoulders and head lift as a result of an *abdominal* contraction.

Variation

To add obliques, raise one shoulder toward the opposite knee, keeping the shoulder back. (In other words, don't collapse the torso as you twist.)

Abdominal Exercises

REMINDER:

REMINDER:

1. Curl and uncurl spine, rather than lifting a straight, stiff torso

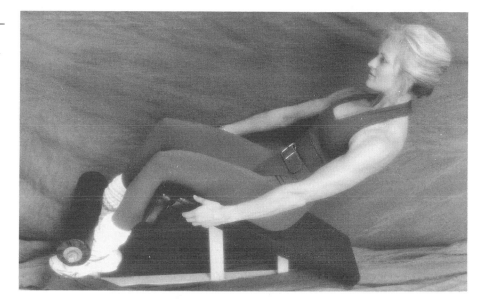

Abdominal Exercises

Exercise 41   Good Old Crunches

BASIC EXERCISE   As basic as it gets. Crunches focus the work in the upper portion of the abdominals. There's much debate about "upper" and "lower" abs, since the fibers on this muscle are all connected and theoretically, therefore, are all activated in any one move. However, I certainly feel this much more in the "upper fibers." It's also more effective after working the "lower" portion first.

Movement   Put your feet on the floor or on a bench—or lie on the floor and drape your legs up across the bench. Try pressing your heels down into the floor or bench. This contracts and virtually paralyzes the hip flexors to guarantee this is all abdominal work. Place your hands behind your head or on your chest.

Drawing with the weight   Lift your head and shoulders off the floor or bench from 3 o'clock to 2 o'clock.

Safety tips   Keep your lower back on the floor or bench. Lift and lower your shoulders with control. Rest your head in your hands, and focus through your legs, rather than up at the ceiling (to decrease neck tension). Avoid yanking on your neck.

Targeted muscles   Rectus abdominus.

Main moving joints   Vertebrae in the middle back.

Function   This muscle helps flex the spine. When you add a twist, activating obliques, it mimics all the side bends and twists that occur in daily life.

Aesthetics   This helps chisel in the top two sections of the "six-pack."

Tricks of the trade   Think of this as an isometric. Hold the contraction and then lift higher and hold, lift higher and hold, etc., until you can't lift anymore.

No cheating   No zooming through these just to get them done. Go slowly into that good set.

Visualization   Imagine you've got an apple tucked under your chin to keep your head and neck in alignment.

Variation   Raise the opposite *shoulder* (not the elbow) to work the obliques. Also, to activate a larger range of motion, simultaneously combine crunches with reverse curls (i.e., lift the opposite shoulder and hip).

Abdominal Exercises

REMINDERS:

1. Rest head in hands
2. Lift shoulders off floor
3. Concentrate on contracting abdominals, rather than just curling spine

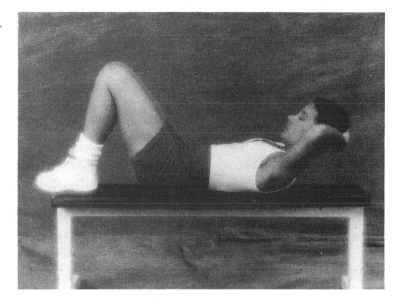

Stretches

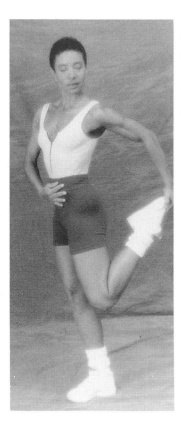

REMINDER: To blend both the hard and soft, strength and flexibility, stretch between sets. Match the working muscle with the appropriate stretch. Hold all stretches for at least 10 seconds, and every time you exhale, let your muscles lengthen even more. Be careful not to bounce or pull too hard on your joints.

1. Quad stretch. Stand on a soft, supporting knee, balancing through the center of your foot. Pull the other heel toward the buttocks.

2. Hip flexor. Lie on the edge of a bench so that your leg hangs down towards the floor. Pull the opposite knee to your chest.

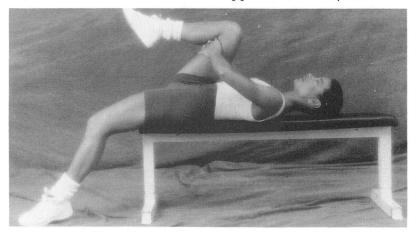

3. Hamstring. Lie on the floor or on a bench. Extend your foot to the ceiling, bending the knee slightly. Gently pull the leg towards your chest. Put the other foot on the floor for back support.

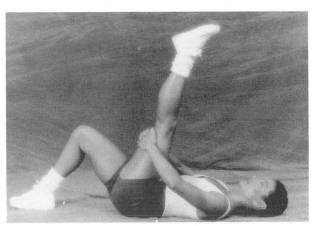

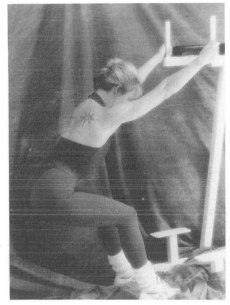

4. Lower back. Hold onto a fixed pole (something you can't pull over). Round your lower back and lean away from the pole.

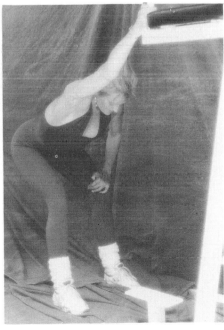

5. Lat stretch. Same as above with one arm only. Keep your lower back in neutral. Stretch from the waist to under the armpit.

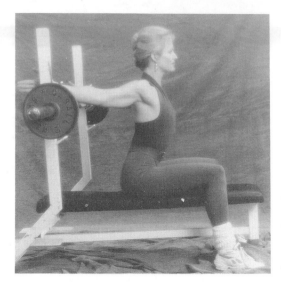

6. Chest. Sit or stand between two poles or in a doorway. Hold on and lean your torso slightly forward.

7. External rotators. Hold onto a towel behind your back. Pull down for external rotators.

8. Internal rotators. Pull up on a behind-the-back towel for internal rotators.

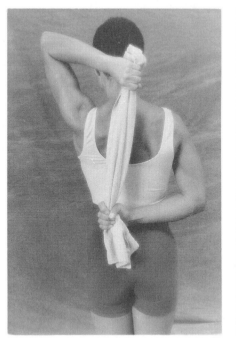

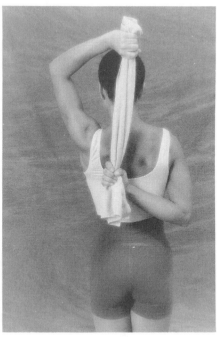

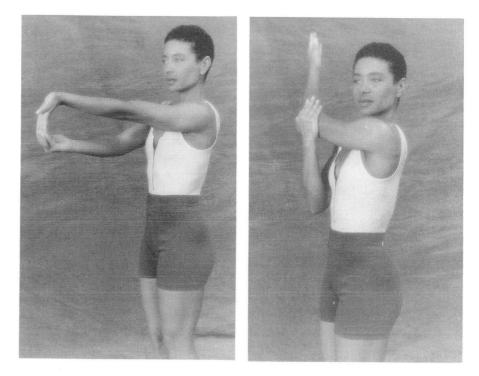

9. Biceps. Pull your fingers down towards the floor. If you have "hyperflexible" elbows, don't pull your arm beyond straight.

10. Triceps, shoulder. Cross your arm over your chest, holding the elbow.

11. Abdominals. Lie on the floor, extending your arms overhead. Let your lower back arch slightly. Stretch from fingers to toes.

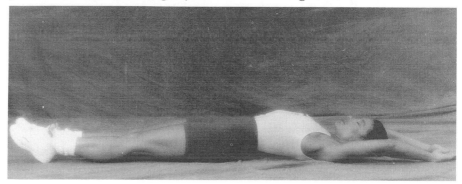

Sample Workouts

IN THE BEGINNING, it helps to keep a notebook for your workouts. This not only serves as a record of your quickly multiplying strength, but is also a good learning tool so you become familiar with the names of exercises. Write exercises according to this universal formula: Name, sets × reps × amount of weight.

In all but the first beginner workouts, I've excluded writing in the weight, since that changes for everyone. Typical weights are given for the beginner workouts so you have an idea how to write the formula and so you can see where many people actually begin. (These are average weights for many novice women.) Please don't let your ego suffer if you must do less. Also, understand that different pieces of equipment feel "light or heavy." Thirty pounds on one cable machine or leg extension, for example, might feel like 50 on another.

Be sure to warm up before every workout, doing about 5 minutes of cardiovascular movement to raise your body temperature and "get the kinks out." Follow that with some light stretches and your first warmup set using light weight, which basically doesn't count as part of the workout.

Beginner Workouts

FULL BODY WORKOUT #1

Alternate between workouts 1 and 2 (see "Sample Beginner Weekly Menu," page 204). Workout 1 starts with higher reps, lighter weight on the first set. The second set is shorter and heavier, to build strength. Workout 2 stays at the same weight, adding more reps on the second set to improve muscular endurance. (NOTE: When you do 2 or 3 sets per exercise you can abbreviate the formula this way: "Leg press 2×15 - 20×70 - 90. The first numbers of each hyphenated set refer to the first set, the second to the second set, and so on.)

Warmup—5 minutes stationary bike

Warmup stretches—lower back, quad, hamstring and hip flexor

Sit-back squats	2×15
Leg press	$2 \times 15 - 10 \times 70 - 90$
Calf press (on leg press)	$2 \times 25 - 15 \times 70 - 90$
Leg extension	$2 \times 12 - 10 \times 20 - 30$
Lying hamstring curls	$2 \times 15 - 12 \times 20 - 30$
Bench press, free bar or Smith	$2 \times 12 - 8 \times 20 - 30$
Lat pull-down to chest	$2 \times 12 - 8 \times 40 - 50$
Shoulder press	$2 \times 12 - 8 \times 5 - 10$
Barbell biceps curl	$2 \times 12 - 8 \times 15 - 20$
Triceps press-down	$2 \times 12 - 8 \times 30 - 40$
Reverse curls for abs	$2 \times 10 - 20$

Cool-down stretches: Abdominal, lower back, lat, chest

FULL BODY WORKOUT #2

Warmup—five minutes stair machine or treadmill walking

Warmup stretches—same as above

Warmup set—sit-back squats	1×15
Smith machine squats	$2 \times 10 \text{-} 15$
In-place lunges, no weight or Smith	$2 \times 12 \text{-} 15$
Standing hamstring curls (machine or ankle weights)	$2 \times 12 \text{-} 15 \times 5$
Hip extension	$2 \times 12 \text{-} 15 \times 20$
Inner thigh cable	$2 \times 10 \text{-} 15 \times 5$
Leg raise on decline	$2 \times 10 \text{-} 15$
Seated calf raise	$2 \times 15 \text{-} 20 \times 40$
Seated cable row	$2 \times 10 \times 15 \times 40$
Chest flyes	$2 \times 8 \text{-} 12 \times 5$
Lateral raises—shoulders	$2 \times 8 \text{-} 12 \times 5$
Dumbbell biceps curls	$2 \times 8 \text{-} 12 \times 8$
Reverse curls for abs	$2 \times 10 \text{-} 20$
Crunches	$2 \times 10 \text{-} 20$

Cool-down stretches: same as above, adding biceps, shoulders/triceps

SAMPLE BEGINNER WEEKLY MENU

Monday: Workout #1

Tuesday: Aerobics only—aerobics class, brisk walk or run

Wednesday: Workout #2

Thursday: Aerobics only—swim, walk or aerobics class

Friday: Workout #1

Saturday: Water exercise, yoga or walk—healing, active rest

Sunday: Off

Monday: Begin cycle with Workout #2

Continue cycle for 6 weeks to 3 months of muscle "initiation"

Intermediate Workouts

BACK AND BICEPS

Warmup—rower, ergometer for 5 minutes

Warmup stretches—lower back and lat stretch

Warmup set—Straight arm press-downs	2 × 8 - 12 using light weight
Lat pull-downs to chest	2 × 8 - 12
Seated cable row	2 × 8 - 12
One-arm row	2 × 8 - 12
Lower back hyperextension	2 × 8 - 12
Barbell biceps curl	2 × 8 - 12
Incline cable curl	2 × 8 - 12
Reverse curls for abs	2 × 15 - 30

Cool-down stretches—lat, lower back and biceps

LEGS

Warmup—stair machine, 5 minutes

Warmup stretches—quad, hamstring and hip flexor

Warmup set—Leg extension	2 × 10 - 15
Leg press	2 × 15
Smith Machine lunges	2 × 10 - 15
Prone hamstring curl	2 × 10 - 15
Hip extension with cable	2 × 15
Standing calf raise	2 × 15 - 25

Cool-down stretches—same as above, plus lower back

CHEST, SHOULDERS, TRICEPS

Warmup—bike 5 minutes

Warmup stretches—chest stretch and external rotator

Warmup set—Bench press	1 × 15 × light weight
Bench press with bar or Smith—flat or incline	2 × 8 - 12
Dumbbell press—flat or incline	2 × 8 - 12
Cable crossovers or dumbbell flyes	2 × 8 - 12
Front cable raise	2 × 8 - 12
Lateral raise	2 × 8 - 12
Triceps extension	2 × 8 - 12
Press-downs	2 × 8 - 12
Reverse curls for abs	2 × 30
Crunches	2 × 30

Cool-down stretches—chest, shoulders, lower back and abs

SAMPLE INTERMEDIATE WEEKLY MENU

Monday: Back, biceps, abs

Tuesday: Aerobics only—stair machine, intervals 30–45 minutes, run or brisk walk

Wednesday: Legs

Thursday: Aerobics only—water exercise or hour-long hike

Friday: Chest, shoulders, triceps, abs

Saturday: Aerobics class

Sunday: Yoga, water exercise or nothing at all!

Advanced Workouts

BACK, REAR DELT, ABS

Warmup—rowing ergometer, 5 minutes

Warmup stretch—lat and lower back

Warmup sets—Straight arm press-downs	3 × 8 - 12
Lat pull-down to chest	3 × 12 - 6
One-arm row	3 × 12 - 6
Seated cable row	3 × 12 - 6
Lower back hyperextensions	3 × 15
Rear delt, cable pullback	3 × 8 - 12
Reverse curls for abs and obliques	3 × 30
Cool-down stretches—triceps/shoulder, lat, lower back, abs	

QUADS, INNER THIGH, CALVES

Warmup—bike 5 minutes

Warmup stretches—quad and hip flexor

Warmup set—Leg extension	1 × 15 × light weight
Leg extension	3 × 12 - 8
Hack squat	3 × 20 - 8
Lunges, rear foot elevated	2 - 3 × 15
Inner thigh cables	2 - 3 × 12 - 15
Standing calf raise	3 × 15 - 25
Seated calf raise	3 × 15 - 25
Cool-down stretches—quad, hip flexor, lower back, standing calf stretch	

CHEST AND SHOULDERS

Warmup—bike 5 minutes

Warmup stretches—chest, external rotator, lower back

Warmup sets—Bench press	2 × 12 × light weight
Flat bench press (bar or dumbbell)	3 × 10 - 6
Incline dumbbell press	3 × 10 - 6
Incline dumbbell flyes or cable crossovers	3 × 12 - 8
Shoulder press	3 × 12 - 8
Lateral raise	3 × 12 - 8
Lying cable front raise	3 × 12 - 8
Super-set lying half uprights	3 × 12 - 8
Cool-down stretches—chest, rotators, lower back	

BUTTOCKS, HAMSTRINGS, OUTER THIGH

Warmup—stair machine, 5 minutes

Warmup stretches—hamstring, hip flexor

Warmup set—Smith Machine squat	1 × 12 × light weight
Smith Machine squats	3 × 25 - 8
Reverse hack squat	3 × 25 - 15
Hip extension with cables	2 × 15
Standing hamstring curl	3 × 15 - 12
Prone hamstring curl	3 × 15 - 8
Smith Machine "stiff" deadlifts	2 × 15
Decline leg raise	3 × 15 - 20
Calf press in leg press machine	3 × 25 - 15
Cool-down stretches—hamstring, hip flexor, lower back, standing calf stretch	

ARMS AND ABS

Warmup—brisk walk 5 minutes

Warmup stretches—lower back, biceps, triceps/shoulder

Warmup set—Dumbbell or barbell biceps curl	1 × 15
Dumbbell or barbell biceps curl	3 × 12 - 6
Incline cable curl	2 × 12 - 8
Preacher curl	2 × 12 - 8
Suicides on decline	3 × 12 - 8
One-arm extension	2 × 12 - 8
One-arm cable press-down	2 × 12 - 8
Rollbacks	3 × 30

Cool-down stretches—biceps, triceps/shoulder, lower back, abs

SAMPLE ADVANCED WEEKLY MENU

Monday: Back, rear delt, abs
  Aerobics—easy bike, 30 minutes

Tuesday: Quads, inner thigh, calves
  Aerobics—brisk walk, stairs, light run, 30 to 40 minutes

Wednesday: Chest, shoulders
  No aerobics

Thursday: Active rest—swim, walk, stretch

Friday: Buttocks, hamstrings, outer thigh
  Aerobics—easy bike, 30 minutes

Saturday: Arms, abs
  Aerobics—stair machine, intervals, 30–40 minutes

Sunday: Active or total rest

Part Four

The Rewards of Practice: Heart, Mind & Future

Transcendental Repetitions

"Framing"

After dwelling in the land of geometry, physics, leverage and bio-mechanics, it's refreshing to return to the mind, the great command control center that colors your experience. By now it should be obvious that there's more to training than "just doing it," more involved than "Okay, lift, lower." You can measure weight, reps, speed, distance, body fat and size, but you can't measure intensity, focus, play, pleasure, confusion, frustration, breakthrough. The heart, mind and soul can't fit into equations like $3 \times 10 \times 15$. But they can help guide you to where you yearn to go. You have the power to make your workout hard, soft, cerebral, intuitive, artistic, even transcendental so that it delivers you right into or out of yourself, whichever you desire.

All you need to do is to search out those moments that free your spirit from its cage and follow that instinct to breathe, move and play. Build a mood in your mind and a fire under your butt, and when the mood fizzles and the fire burns low, change moods, tempo, paint a new picture in your mind or stop. You've got all the tools you need to recreate the experience for yourself every day and moment by moment. Sometimes you'll get lost in it; the mind will drift and movement will seem to take over. Other times, you'll have to steer the craft with conscious thought and unexpectedly change course. You are both the vessel and the wind.

Forget guilt, calories, social pressure and the "need" to look a certain way. Tap into the *significance* of what you're doing. This is your sacred time to reconnect. You will begin to find that there is nothing truly different about your life in motion from your life standing still. The same issues that you encounter on a larger scale apply in tangible form to your movement life as well. Look for the themes and weave them like a thread through every action. This helps you "frame" your activity within a larger scope and gives it meaning. Explore:

- Balance—Delve into the subtleties of how your weight shifts from the ball of the foot to the heel. Study the effect on your bones, your carriage, the way your movement is hindered or freed up—the same effect on a house, if the foundation were to suddenly shift. Or hold a weight in each hand and practice the geometrical art of symmetrical motion, one half of you perfectly mirroring the other—even if, when you look very closely, it doesn't.

- Humility—Pay homage to the smallest weights and/or the tiniest muscles, the ones no one can see. Block out other people so you can set all comparisons aside. Enter the land of the beginner, even if you aren't one, and walk through a movement as if you've never done it before. Take any exercise and break it down to its minute parts so you learn to respect the requirements of one "perfect" rep—even if you're a long way off.

- Finesse—Practice the art of detail. Take up the master's chisel and etch in the outer edge of a particular muscle, even if the inner part isn't fully there yet. Notice the fine points of a turned-out leg or a slightly bent arm and see how that affects where you feel a particular movement. Mine the infinite source of variations and become the master craftswoman.

- Power—Cut back to the sheer simplicity of muscle and bone in action. Find the safest and most efficient way to hoist a load, doing away with all extraneous motion.

- Trust in yourself/Evolution—Focus on the exercises that were hard in the beginning and are now a smooth part of your repertoire. Observe how some once-dreaded movements have evolved into favorites, weak spots into new strengths. Do them once again, with your hard-earned ability, and acknowledge how far you've come.

When the sameness of a routine dulls the sharp edges of your wits, make up games:

- Do exercises that only work one limb at a time—the traditional ones: leg extensions, hamstring curls, dumbbell curls, one-arm press-downs for triceps—and the nontraditional: leg presses, regular and reverse hack squats, cable crossovers. See how many exercises you can "convert" to one limb only.

- One-minute drills—Use a stopwatch with an alarm and time yourself to make sure each set lasts for 60 seconds (hint—pace yourself; it's a long time). Make sure your rests don't last longer.

- Practice lifting without showing an ounce of strain. Keep your face calm and make no noise.

- Commit yourself not to take up time by talking between sets or looking around the room.

- Create a workout as a "performance piece." Give it a clear beginning, middle and end. Choose exercises as a painter chooses colors, a writer words. Fit them together in a way that is pleasing even if it doesn't make total sense. Don't be afraid to break the mold or, if something isn't working, to move onto something else.

There's no end to the ways you can "frame" your workouts, no limit to the imagination. As you slip into your self-made world, freeing your wild spirit, taking care of your tender soul, generating new sources of power in your being, you aren't, despite what others may think, simply involved in a highly selfish act. Your actions affect others, even when they seem private. You may be striding down the street with arms pumping, tuned into your own private rhythms. A woman looks out her window and realizes she's forgotten to take care of herself today and heads out for a walk. Or you've just gotten started weight training consistently. Your body has just begun to change but your manner is different. A friend notices a new calm, a substance in your being, and she want this too, and joins the gym. You may weight train in your living room and hike alone on deserted hilltops, but you aren't really alone. So do millions of others, more and more women all the time. Your participation expands the consciousness by one more soulful mind. Do not stop, because you are needed. There's so much more to be done, so many more women who long to fill their lives with such feelings. Your actions lift others up.

Ground and Center

Taking yourself into a playful state isn't just automatic. Running from the car or your job right into a workout doesn't exactly create the right atmosphere for this opening. Yes, you can start moving and find yourself suddenly "awake at the wheel." But it's better to grant yourself a few moments to "ground and center," either before or during a warmup. Take off the mask and create a clearing, prepare the canvas, set the stage for magic.

Like a pilot in a cockpit, don't take off until you run through a simple checklist. The list needn't be as long as this. But when you ask yourself questions, be sure to listen for the answers. Some examples:

- How am I today?

- Who am I today?

- Is there an emotion charging through my heart that I need to take into consideration—and use in the workout?

- Do I hurt anywhere, physically?

- Is there a move I should avoid or an area to grant special care?

- What body parts am I working today?

- What was the last workout I did for those muscles?

- What angles, weights, exercises or rep ranges haven't I used for a while?

- What's a good warmup for those body parts?

- How much time do I have?

- How can I use the time most effectively?

- Do I want to start with pressing moves (those straight-line motions) that use several joints and muscles at once—so I can lift heavier first?

- Or do I want to start with more isolation moves (those arcing motions), so I can "pre-exhaust" my muscles first and later won't need to press so much weight?

- Am I doing aerobics today?

- If so, when? What type?

- Is there a theme today?

- A game to play to pepper up my routine?

- Do I need to "zip myself into my idealized self"?

- Or am I on my own today?

- Am I ready to begin?

Journey into the Soul of a Transcendental Set

In a perfect world, each set should represent a philosophy, a total approach boiled down to its essence, a magnum opus as expressed in Haiku. Every set, in fact every rep, is an opportunity to put theory into practice and come alive in the present. Yet, since that doesn't always happen, training is very forgiving, too; for when one opportunity is lost, another follows on its heels.

You might suppose that a "transcendental" set would require no thinking at all, that the mind and motion would be so artfully entwined, there'd be no room for conscious thought, just a kind of at-one-ness. Yes. But to get to that place takes practice, practice, practice and an almost subterranean level of scanning and quick decision-making that is virtually nonstop. It all happens at the speed of thought—much faster than it takes to read these words. But if you examined the thought process at slow r.p.m.'s, it might sound something like this:

- You quickly, roughly plan the whole workout—the order of exercises, equipment, any particular exercise that requires your greatest attention; the bench press, for example. You leave room for variables—machines being used, etc. You identify the general flavor of movement today to suit your mood.

- You choose an exercise and quickly double-check to make sure that's a sound choice. Does it match your needs? Does it put you at risk? If it doesn't work, choose another. If it does work, plan the variations for each set. Are you starting light, working up to heavy, or starting heavier and ending with high reps? Or perhaps doing something altogether different? If you could chart your intensity on a graph, how would it curve?

- You prepare your equipment, adjusting the seat if necessary, carrying free weights over to the bench, resting them on the floor.

- You place yourself on the bench and, if using free weights, roll them into place in a way that uses momentum to get them up safely. You make sure your grip is even, placement symmetrical.

- You double-check alignment, sensing the imaginary vertical pole running through the midline and the horizontals through the neck, shoulders, hips, knees and feet.

- You focus on a spot right in front of you, soften your vision to everything else around, calm your breathing.

- You take a moment to "run" energy through your body—not too much, just a sense of prickly heat, a beam of light, a gentle hum.

- You begin the movement by tracing clean lines or round arcs with the weights or your body, precisely marking the beginning and end of each movement.

- At the "top" of each contraction, you squeeze the muscle, holding on to the floodgate of fullness for as long as you can.

- As you lower the weight, you pause for a moment at the bottom, as if putting in a comma between phrases.

- In a full stretched position, you "absorb" the weight into your muscles, let them suck it up like a sponge.

- Before starting the next rep, you take inventory over muscles and joints, and if they're "off," compose and then continue.

- As the fire builds in the muscles, you feel your heart race, your neck muscles clamp down, the nerves, joints and lactic acid signaling the body beginning to go into all-out protest.

- But you are practiced at this, breathe, gather strength and open your nerves to the sensation because this is where the strength takes hold.

- The fire burns. You cannot stay here long. The form is going. So you quickly put down your weight in an artful half moment, pick up lighter weights and continue.

- The new weight feels light for a rep or two and then absurdly heavy, a joke, an insult.

- But you play with it, add a slight pulse, a hold, another deep breath, milking everything possible from the motion.

- Involuntary movements start to take over. Limbs shake. Your foot taps for some odd reason you have never been able to figure out. You're no longer in total control. The mind is saying, "That's enough," but you know your body can do at least two more reps, keeping integrity intact.

- So you take a deep breath and override the sensation with your will. You tell your muscles, "yes," policing your form like a prison guard because you know that when you force your will (because you may be a willful person) you sometimes go too far, lose sensitivity and tempt the danger. But paying attention to form lets you know when you've gone too far. And the form is going . . .

- You can no longer continue without cheating, so you just hold the weight, hanging out here on the edge, biting down in the jaw, coaxing one more fiber, and the moment stretches out like a desert.

- You want to drop the weight and scream but instead, lower it with the exquisite sensitivity of a mother laying down the head of her newborn. You bring it to a visible stop, put a period on the sentence, hold it for a moment. Done.

- When you rack the weight, you put it back with the same care with which you did the set. What a waste it would be to chuck all your careful motion now and throw a muscle.

- The pain scurries away like a forgotten dream on a busy morning.

- You step away from the exercise, look back for a moment to appreciate the work you've just done.

- Those full, hot, fatigued muscles surrender to the reward of a long, luxurious stretch. You rest, regroup.

- And when you're ready, begin again.

The Pleasure of Partnering

When you work out alone, such epiphanies are private. When you work out with a partner, the experience is shared. As in any supportive relationship, the sum total of one plus one equals far more than two. Between two there is an invisible third—that thing called "us" and the mysterious surges of strength that come when someone simply stands behind offering physical, verbal or even silent support. This is the common but magical force that is generated by two people helping each other get stronger. Intimate bonds are built on this. (I married my best training partner.)

As in life, training partnerships work best when the two people are linked by mutual desire. It's not so important that strength be equal— but that the approach be compatible and both contribute. When one person struts around, showing off, and the other feels weak and uncoordinated, the relationship is imbalanced and it's no fun for the "humbled" person. Chances are good such a partnership won't last. As in a marriage, two people have to put in equal portions of intent. Unlike a trainer/client relationship, in which there's an obvious leader and follower, training partners work best when they're at about the same level of knowledge and desire.

Working with a partner is a close exchange, based on trust. You move into each other's experience, reveal your funny faces and weaknesses, let someone into your world and enter theirs, so that both of you may be assisted, corrected, coached. When you lift heavy weight, you have to know you can count on your partner and provide the same in return.

It's very annoying when a partner's attention wanders, especially at a critical moment with a bar suspended over your head. It's equally annoying when he or she helps too much, practically doing the lift for you, lacking the sensitivity for an appropriate touch. Helping too little is dangerous. Helping too much doesn't make either person strong.

A Good Spot

Good partnering in the weight room is like partnering on the dance floor. You need to develop the "feel" for when to lead and when to follow, when to move together and when to solo. Clear communication helps. Lifters should:

- Say how many reps they expect to do without help,

- Say how many more reps they want to do *with* help,

- Alert their partner if they need assistance racking and unracking the weight,

- Specify what sort of spot they want—for instance, on pull-ups, do they want to be held under the knees or around the waist; on a squat, around the waist or hips?

Spotters should:

- Put themselves in a safe position—with a wide, semi squat-type stance, making sure *they're* not doing the work or straining any muscles, particularly when spotting bench presses, pull-ups or squats. Use a strong, slightly contracted lower back. Don't round.

- Spot under the elbows; on exercises such as a dumbbell press, don't lift the weights.

- Make sure to push the person straight up on pull-ups, not up and back or up and forward.

- Be there for every second of every rep.

- Use a light touch—adding a bit more help as required. For instance, on a bench press or pull-down, simply assist with one finger. As it gets harder, add two fingers and then three or the whole hand. If the spotter has to work too hard, the lifter has no business using so much weight.

- Show the lifter how much additional force was added, by demonstrating on their arm the amount of lift or saying, "I lifted about 2 pounds."

- Avoid getting in the way of the motion.

- Try not to stand directly in front of the mirror. Spot from behind.

- Use supportive verbal cues, such as, "That's it, keep your shoulders down" rather than negatives, such as, "Don't lift your shoulders."

Both partners should tell each other the sort of verbal and physical support they like. For instance, I respond well to positive reinforcement, such as, "Good form." Even if my form is falling apart, I'll work to correct it, as if I want to live up to that person's good impression of me. I hate being told, "Come on, dig" or "Work." That elicits an immediate negative response from me. The devil in me thinks, "I *am* digging and working. What are *you* doing?" especially when that other person has no idea what's going on in my body or mind or has rushed up with an unsolicited spot, to rescue the little lady in distress.

Gym Etiquette

With all this emphasis on "mindfulness" and awareness to the extreme, it's out of line to treat the equipment or others with no care. Please be sure to avoid:

- leaving plates loaded on a machine

- banging plates with every rep

- leaving sweat on a bench

- hogging a machine someone else wants to use. Ask if they'd like to "work in."

Like good kids, remember to share, take good care of the toys and put them away.

Working Out with "Difficult" Emotions

EMOTIONS SEEM TO RIDE IN on the wind without warning. But when an emotional elephant flies through the door and lands on your chest, it's sometimes tough just to go *out*, let alone slog through a workout. Deep, "difficult" emotions and workouts aren't an obvious mix. The logical thinking is, "I already hurt. Who needs more pain?" No wonder people give up on exercise just when they need it most.

Others use workouts as a way to avoid bigger feelings. It's much easier to tolerate physical discomfort than the soul-shaking, slow-moving emotional issues that seize the heart.

There's a third choice, however. You can *use* your emotions to get a better workout and use your workouts to experience feelings in a different way. When you let your sadness, anger, fear, or some other emotion play itself out through your movements, something very interesting happens. You may feel stirred up, touched, slowed down, yanked out of habitual thinking and put in a slightly altered state. You get to "see" your feelings in action. If you harness these emotions wisely and use them to your advantage, you create something life-sustaining and beautiful from the ashes. The phoenix rises. Emotions also tend to move out much faster when you give them room to be. You may even have your best workouts on these days and make important discoveries.

You certainly don't have to manufacture a false enthusiasm to get yourself moving or cut off your feelings for the time it takes you to work out. It's much easier to go with your natural flow and move as a "whole" person.

Try to boil down all your feelings into one word, as in "I feel sad" or "afraid." Whenever you change that phrase to "I feel *that*" followed by a slew of words (such as "I feel that I need to be appreciated more and . . . blah, blah"), you've entered the land of your head. Keep it simple and you come from your heart. Once you identify the emotion, then you can work with it.

Each feeling seems to dictate its own laws of motion. You may or may not find that these work for you. But if you want to give them a try, I suggest you reread the appropriate section on days when the feelings hit hard.

Sadness / Depression

Sadness and depression add weight to your bones, density to your flesh and effort to all movements. You hunch over, shuffle along, barely lift your feet. You seem to have gained pounds and years, lost stature. You might actually shrink a few inches, because posture's the first thing to go.

Sadness is a slightly more active state than depression. Depression is more of a black hole, an absence of feeling, barometric pressure dropping to zero. At least with sadness there are rainstorms, tears. But with depression, it's tough just to move. Both emotions, however, can heighten sensuality, make sad songs sadder, the blues bluer, old memories more bitter than sweet. The difficult part is overcoming inertia and simply getting out of bed. Habit is useful here. Once in motion, you might discover that you move with a different sort of grace, feel compassion for similar creatures, notice wounded birds, limping dogs, downcast people sitting motionless on park benches. You move through the world in a blur, sensitive to loud noises, quick actions, as if permanently hungover.

This is a time to travel slowly, hold back a bit, treat yourself with extra softness—and put your primary focus on posture. This is not a time to exert too strenuously, bother with counts, heart rates or matching past achievements. Hard as this may sound, this is a time to feel. Sadness and depression humble. To compare your moves today with those on other days might simply make you more depressed. This is an opportunity to throw out the usual, abandon expectation and nurture yourself in the sheer act of motion—however subtle it may be.

You can't force yourself out of it, so you might as well sway to its bluesy melody. It will lift on its own. Movement might even help cook it away. But it's best to be in slow motion, pull tiny victories from the smallest details, let every silky movement become a caress and settle in for long, static stretches. Make sure that you dress warmly. Depression breeds inertia. Being cold makes movement tougher.

This might also be a good day to head to the pool (if the water's warm) and leave your dead weight on land.

Vulnerable / Hurting

Sometimes, as you travel from grief to acceptance, sickness to wellness, victim to victor, your very nerve endings seem to end just outside your skin. Manufacturing a false cheerfulness takes a lot of energy and feels ridiculous. And yet, walking through the world feeling vulnerable is like walking down a crowded street without clothes. You need a certain amount of camouflage to survive, although armoring your heart isn't the answer, either. Owning the vulnerability in all its naked glory, even if it's just your own precious secret, will give you a source of strength no one else needs to see.

Vulnerability will most likely center in the chest. The back rounds forward to protect a fragile heart. This is a good day to work the chest, fill the area with strength and heat, do a little "open heart surgery." You might feel exposed in the posture but others will only notice that you look better. You can still hide your wounded self even behind good posture, if that's your wish.

It helps to stay in continual motion. Beware of resting too long, letting your mind drift. Movements that require mental skills, with tricky, challenging counts demand more of your attention, keep your mind engaged and take the energy up.

This is not the day for trying new sports, breaking records in the weight room or trying hang gliding. If you're vulnerable in your emotions, you're more likely to be vulnerable in your body, too. You should respect tender spots and avoid careless moves that could blossom into injury.

Fear

There are many shades of fear, from nervous excitement to paranoia. Many emotions, such as guilt, hate and anxiety, actually boil down to fear. Even falling in love or experiencing a positive change can make you afraid. One unifying characteristic of fear is that it's usually about the past or future, seldom about what's happening right now. Fear has been called the opposite of love. I believe this is so. In a loving state, you're open, forgiving, present, patient and aware. In fear, you're contracted, not trusting, rigid. The old Fight or Flight Syndrome takes hold of the body, preparing you to strike out or flee. Your breathing gets shallow. Your neck and shoulders tighten. You're ready to bite and operate more off "lizard brain" survival skills than higher consciousness. There's nothing wrong with this. Everyone goes through it. But it's only part of who you are.

Before beginning a workout, take even more time to "ground and center," breathe. When you're afraid, the mind is in charge. Breathing leads you out of your mind and into your body. When the body is calm, the mind follows. Come back to the present, taking note of your surroundings, the pleasant details of the room or outside. Notice how safe you are right now.

When you move aerobically, fear can make jackrabbit steps of your movements, give you speed, a jittery sort of acceleration you can use to your advantage. With fear to burn, it's a good opportunity to do intervals—a minute at a hard pace, followed by two to three minutes at a moderate pace, repeating the cycle several times. A workout like that could deliver you back to normal faster than you might realize.

Working with weights gives you a special opportunity to confront and conquer fear. Believe it or not, it often helps to do something that really scares you—more weight on the leg press, for instance, or a personal best on the bench press—just as long as you're warmed up and have a spotter. Your goal should be simple. Unrack the weight, hold it for a second and rack it again, approaching fear with intelligence and caution. When you're confident you can at least hold the weight, *then* try a quarter-rep and rack it again, then a half-rep, full rep, etc. This way you break it down into tiny, manageable, nonthreatening pieces. Fear then turns to victory and profound satisfaction.

Fear often centers in the shoulders, neck and jaw. Stretching out these areas helps release residual tension.

Anger

Anger can bubble and build silently under the surface like molten lava. It can surprise, erupt, scorch anything in its path. Anger, like fear, tightens muscles, jerks movements and quickens breathing. It also generates lots of power—some good, some destructive.

When you're angry, you have more energy. It's easy to throw things in a rage and hurt yourself (or somebody else). But if anger is used wisely, if you hold back just a little and smolder rather than burn, you can bring the anger under control and also use the energy wisely. Tempered anger can inspire a great workout.

When motions become sloppy and frantic, pull back and think, plan strategies or even revenge. Just make sure the opponent is the weight, not yourself or anyone else. With anger, you can punctuate each movement with a boxer's jab and use precision to push yourself harder, lift heavier, reach for new personal bests.

When anger comes after depression, energy surges. It's the active force rearing its head. It's also the dominant emotion used by teams and coaches to build motivation. But too often it's the only emotion that some (mostly male) athletes know how to use—and so they generate it even when it isn't there, just to get the rush. Simply feeling good and centered can probably create the same sort of power, without the distraction of sloppiness, inappropriate aggression and careening out of balance.

Tired

Tired obviously isn't an emotion; yet it's worth mentioning here. When you're tired, the mind/muscle link is a little slow, sometimes nonexistent, but not beyond hope.

When you work out aerobically, you need to double your warmup time and stay ten, rather than five, minutes in the easy-to-moderate zone, even hold yourself back so you itch to go faster. Listening to the most uplifting music you can find sometimes pulls you right out of tired. If not, it's a good time for an "LSD"—a "long, slow and distance" workout for 45 minutes to an hour, in the low end of your target heart zone.

In a weight workout, this is a good time to take a new look at old exercises, drop weights by half and do 10-second reps. Treat yourself to a "humbling workout," an opportunity to abandon all expectations, ask for nothing, expect nothing and realize that nothing is required. With no expectation, there's no disappointment. Everything you do after that is a bonus. Thus, you're free to play around and stop whenever you want.

This is also another good day to head to the pool for the rejuvenating power of water.

Rest

Some days the forces are greater than you are. The weights are too heavy, feelings too thick, gravity too dense. Your heart may be raw, your mind slow, and no matter what you do, you just can't get started. When that's the case, don't force it. What you may need instead is a passive stretch. Simply put yourself into different positions and let gravity do the work. Surrender. Or forget it altogether and meditate, daydream, curl up, read, watch a movie or go to sleep. A day like this is often followed by one of clarity, power and ease.

The Power Zone

I N THIS LAND OF DISCIPLINE and effort, there is a paradise, a place of ecstasy you might discover by accident and perhaps visit at will. Some athletes call it "the flow" or "being in the zone." In it there's clarity, a sense of extreme focus and control. Yet the energy seems to flow effortlessly, as if you are tapping into a source of power greater than your own. Doubts, fears and obstacles slide away. In their place come confidence, precision, balance. You can almost see what's going to happen right before it does. Whatever the motion, the weight, the ball, your legs go exactly where you want. If there are other players involved, they too go just where you need them, as if you're all tuned to that same station.

Athletic activity isn't the only vessel that takes you there, yet it's one of the most celebrated. It really doesn't matter what you do—sing, write, cook, make love, hammer a nail or drive a car. The zone is the same. Your senses heighten, your abilities sharpen, even rise several notches above the usual. Every movement serves a purpose. Nothing is wasted. The ego slips into the background, diminishing any need to win or prove something. In fact, results become irrelevant. The focus switches to the doing, the exquisite combination of motion, balance, timing, as if you're moving in sync with the universal laws of motion. Games get won this way and records broken. But the real prize is the zone itself. This may, in fact, be our natural state, unimpeded, with no static on the airwaves.

I suspect that most everybody has the ability to experience the zone or at least recognize when someone else is in it. Perhaps this is one reason why there are so many sports fans—for the thrill of living vicariously. (This may also be why there are so many drug addicts—looking for the rush in all the wrong places.) When you watch an athlete perfectly execute a move, your muscles twitch in sympathetic rapture. When one takes a nasty fall, you cringe. Deep down in your instinctual belly, you understand this type of ecstasy (or agony), even if you can't verbalize it or get into this state yourself.

The first time you enter the zone, you probably won't realize it until later because in the moment itself, you're too busy experiencing it. Self-consciousness would upset the flow. But in retrospect, you'll *know* when you were there. You may remember exquisite sensory details—sunlight pouring through trees, the smell of fresh-cut grass, the sound of your breathing, steam rising off your skin, a neon yellow tennis ball hanging in the air for what seems like a minute, energy flooding through your fingertips, an infinite, gushing source. Once you experience this, you'll want to do it again. But it's not so easy.

The question is, how do you get there? I'm not sure it's a journey you make with your will. Yet it isn't a matter of luck, either. It comes after time invested, after developing a certain amount of understanding of the necessary movements. You no longer operate off what I call "level 1" consciousness, reminding yourself of the perfunctories. (Spontaneous breakthrough into the zone seldom happens at the beginner level, though no doubt it has.) The zone seems to occur at least on "level 2" or above, when the movements are natural and ingrained. Mostly it comes from putting yourself into a neutral, receptive state, trusting your ability.

The first time I entered the zone, it happened by accident. For a long time, I wanted the trophy of bench pressing my weight of a hundred and thirty pounds. I had gotten stuck at the plateau of a hundred and because I was younger, felt frustrated. One day, with a spotter, I just decided to put thirty more pounds on the bar (a very stupid thing to do). I was determined just to try it, though I was afraid of getting buried under the weight. So I took a moment to stare at the bar above me and talked myself into a calm state of mind. To my surprise, I unracked the weight myself and it didn't feel as heavy as I thought it would. Then, with no assistance, I ground out three reps. In fact, I seemed to *generate power with every repetition,* as if someone had just injected pure crystallized energy in my veins and pumped Beethoven's "Ode to Joy" at earsplitting volume over the loudspeakers. I was a vessel of strength. Enormous but effortless power poured out of me. And then I jolted out of the dream. My mind said, "Are you crazy? You can't do this," and I got scared. So of course, I immediately fizzled, couldn't even hold the bar anymore and had to be rescued. But I *had* lifted it three times, and that alone was amazing.

Later, I tried another set and couldn't do it—not one rep. Afterwards, I realized that I couldn't do the second set—not because I was fatigued or foolhardy, but because I didn't believe. Even though I'd done it once, doubt had already crept in. My mind said, "Nah," so naturally my body did, too.

Since then, I've learned to believe. Consequently, I hit the zone quite frequently. It isn't such a mysterious state and doesn't have to be tied to breaking records or superhuman surges of strength. Lifting heavy objects, in fact, doesn't have much to do with it at all. I go there using light weight as well. The zone is a state of focus so intense that time seems to bend. All outside distractions disappear and nothing else exists but the moment! My trips into the zone are brief because my sets are relatively brief, though the whole workout can be a kind of zone, with the peaks coming at the height of each set. More practiced yogi/athletes can probably sustain the zone for a longer time, particularly in a nonstop activity such as basketball or running.

I've learned that I can't force myself to get there. I can only create the right conditions. I've hit the zone at the beginning, middle and end of my workouts, when I've been tired, jet-lagged, at all times of the day and in all types of weather. The mind, it seems, has the power to overcome these conditions.

What's consistent each time is setting the mood. Before starting, I stare at a spot in front of me to bring myself "home" and double-check alignment. When I bench press, I wrap my hands around the bar, one at a time, positioning my ring fingers around the clear groove in the rough metal, feeling the cold bar or the heat from the last person who put their hands here. For a moment, I "run" energy through my whole body, as if revving a car. I don't rev too high, as this excites me and wastes energy. I feel relaxed but charged, quiet and ready. I don't give myself a pep talk, because pep talks come when there's doubt. No, I have energy and simply know I can. My focus narrows, and the world around me becomes a blur. All I see is the straight line of the bar, my arms in perfect symmetry. Sometimes I see myself going through the motion before I do it; other times I just enter the moment as fully as I can.

The power zone exists in a place beyond doubt and fear. Mind you, doubt and fear serve important functions, especially as you get older. They're healthy protective modes. But you don't always need to be protected. The safest route into the zone is through an exercise in which you already feel confident. The key, I believe, is trusting yourself.

Ordinary Magic

The power zone is a gift, a blue moon, a rare treat that lifts your heart to the heavens and perhaps even lets you see your life from a lofty perspective, your mate in a golden glow, your children wrapped in the original love that brought them here. It's not an everyday thing—at least not for me. Despite its charms and mystery, it isn't what keeps me training. It's not even my greatest joy. I honestly find more pleasure in the ordinary magic of day-to-day practice. I *like* mundane reality, pushing through PMS, traffic jams, rainy days and my own mental and emotional shortcomings, into the simple majesty of a humbling workout and doing my best for today. It isn't as sexy or glamorous—but that's what makes it even *more* valuable because it's so common and so normal.

Approaching Mastery

I F YOU WANT TO BECOME A MASTER at this or anything, first you must be a seeker. You'll need a certain amount of stubbornness at the pit of your personality, a healthy disregard for pat answers, "experts" and rules written in stone. Although you'll prosper with a solid education and the support of others, you'll also need to press on without them, as a lone wolf on the plain, sometimes running straight through blizzards and blind spots, steering by instinct alone. Don't be afraid to nurture your individual style; honor the inexplicable forces that move you; blend your odd, seemingly unrelated ingredients into an alchemical soup. Don't worry if you feel confused.

As you approach mastery, seek out the simple truths that will be as true tomorrow as they are today. Grow into your gristly strength, solidify your core and your opinions but stay flexible in your method and fluid in your joints. Even masters get crusty. Your mind will keep changing; your body will change also; therefore, your methods must keep changing, as well. But you may find you'll do the same exercises at age 60 or 70 that got you started decades before. They'll continue to get richer and more interesting.

The rewards of mastery are mostly internal and invisible. You may earn trophies, positions of authority, money, admiration, respect—even corporate sponsorship. But don't confuse these with the greatest rewards which grow through humble means—simply showing up day after day, finding joy in the doing, and remembering to treat all fellow travelers with respect. Achieving mastery won't give you permission to swagger, boast, regard anyone as inferior or spill emotions on those in your way. What it will give you is the power of silence. What you know will speak for itself.

As a master you will have learned how to take something difficult and make it look easy. Others will seldom realize the physical and invisible difficulties you may have had to overcome, the emotions that may have bulldozed through self-belief or the mental chatter that every second threatened to snap your concentration in two. What they'll see from the outside is grace in motion, elegance and ease, a self-made person "in the zone." Most likely, they'll think it all came easy. But you'll know better.

Inborn talents are not required. In fact, "talent" often gets in the way because it fuels the ego with expectation that you will "get" something, be rewarded. The ego is useful in that it supplies the drive to excel. But true mastery flourishes when the ego begins to relax after its hard-driven years of youth, when there's no longer such a pressing need to achieve something or be important. Although many of us, myself included, continue to grapple with the hunger for attention well into middle age and beyond, mastery doesn't satisfy this desire. (I sometimes wonder what *does* satisfy it, when and if this hunger will *ever* go away and what indeed caused it to begin with.) Mastery doesn't seem to come until after you no longer need it, when the soul yearns for a substance that grows within. Like a wildflower on a mountaintop, mastery seems to bloom solely for itself; yet its sheer existence touches others.

I have met a few "masters of the iron." It takes a skilled eye to notice them. They wear no distinguishing black belts, have no adoring students bowing and calling them "Sifu." They carry gym bags, wear sweats, grunt and groan like everybody else. Some are my friends; some are legends; some are strangers I've spotted across the gym floor. Whether they are famous champions or "legends in their own minds," they share certain characteristics. They tend to be modest, work out silently and prefer off-hours so they can be left alone. Many slip in and out of the gym almost invisibly, yet you can't help but notice them. They're also the first ones to offer encouragement, support, compliments unsolicited to others just starting on the path. They laugh at the various hip-meisters who claim that muscle-building is no longer in style, ignore faddish training methods claiming to add five pounds of muscle in six weeks and expensive supplements promising "amazing" results. They prefer common sense, slow process, humble progress—and they get better every year.

In the future, there will be more strength-masters—women and men in their forties, fifties, sixties, seventies, eighties, perhaps nineties and beyond. Right now, many are still in the lab experimenting. Most would claim they haven't yet earned the title of "master." Perhaps you will be one of them. Perhaps you already are.

As a master, you make entry into a certain sector of the human race in which sex, race, economic status and brute strength have little meaning. Your shining asset will be your humanity, all the wealth you've created in yourself using your flawed pieces, discipline, imagination and tools at hand. You will be judged not on your physique or brute strength but on the expansiveness of your heart, the pleasure you take in your practice and the personal riches you lovingly pass on to others.

And on into the Future

Though physical strength certainly improves your entire life and decreases your chances of falling prey to injury and disease, it's still no guarantee of shining health. Fitness of any sort has yet to make anyone immortal. No matter how strong and healthy you become, you still won't be immune to the physical tests that increase with age.

Many of you come from high-risk backgrounds, with family histories chock full of heart disease, cancer, Alzheimer's and other debilitating conditions. Or you may have squandered years of your life to various types of drug abuse, self-destruction and neglect. It remains to be seen when and if the effects of *those* days will ever demand reckoning. All you can do to protect yourself from the genetic and self-loaded bullets pointed at your head is everything within your power: eat sensibly, exercise regularly, live a peaceful, loving life, embrace your days, work, relax, trust in the body's ability to heal and regenerate itself, and open yourself to the possibility that you *can* work miracles with your health. You can also be prepared—just in case.

No doubt many of you have watched your parents and grandparents succumb to the cruelties of disease, debilitation and what used to be called "the inevitability of old age." You may have watched their vision, hearing and movement become impaired, seen them become housebound or bedridden and have stood by helplessly as they endured major operations and painful recoveries, witnessing their acts of independence disappear one by one and their spirits slip away. You may have seen them stubbornly reject things that would help them get around— medications, canes, wheelchairs, Seeing Eye dogs, hearing aids, and so forth, as a matter of pride. Although such denial reveals a certain spunk, it mostly demonstrates an unwillingness to deal with the truth. There's that slim hope that if a condition is ignored, it will go away. Ironically, the consequence of such pride is that older people often become more dependent, more isolated and depressed—the ingredients for a downward spiral towards death.

Sometimes bad news from the doctor sets off a desperate, eleventh-hour scramble to radically alter behavior—and sometimes this works. I've seen a lot of older people slash fat from their diet, take up exercise and discover a vigor they didn't even have in their youth. But I've also witnessed others do this only at doctor's orders. There's no fun in that. Their choice has been "change everything or die." Some people need to be brought to their knees before making such changes. There's certainly an easier way.

Habits are hard enough to change at any age, but late in life, habits are solid, the grooves well worn. Although late-in-life changes and "deathbed conversions" do happen all the time, such changes are often too late. All those years of bad living have already taken a toll. A body can't be expected to reverse decades of damage after only a few months or years, no matter how remarkable its ability to heal.

If you were born after 1950, you are part of a privileged generation. With more information about nutrition, exercise and well-being available now than at any time before, you get to live the majority of your life in a healthy way, if you choose. Sadly, even now, many people don't choose. We're all familiar with the excuses—no time, don't feel like it, too difficult to change—and on top of all that, these are toxic times anyway, so why bother? But you *can* take responsibility. You can have your sweat, your muscle, your low-fat foods, your lifestyle that just twenty years ago would have had you branded as a crackpot. The world is not only more accepting, it encourages it, admires it, even if on the outside it expresses jealousy and scorn. It's up to each of you to take a close look at yourself every so often and ask, "Am I really preparing for a long, healthy life?" and if not, "What changes can I make today?"

Unknowns will always dangle at the future's edge. Sickness and injury are fickle, too, sometimes striking the most fit-bodied and sparing those who reveled in self-abuse. Sometimes it seems like a health-crisis lottery—some of us get lucky; others don't. But everyone (at least those outside a war zone) can choose to live at lower risk. Even then, many of you will be tested in some way or another, although it may not happen for years. But when it does, how will *you* respond when the doctor says "surgery," "cancer," or "debilitating disease"? How will you react when age snatches away your abilities, or death creeps down and peers in your window? It's hard to know until you get there.

But you can prepare by building a type of strength that radiates from the core. By continuing to manifest in the physical, the power you have inside, you keep your flames lit, give yourself a potent tool to endure. Such strength lasts for as long as you give it attention. It also has the power to inspire others who recognize its worth.

It's my hope that if and when you are severely tested, your self-built strength can give you the ability to embrace the life you have left, not to mourn the things that get lost. The goal here is to fully inhabit your body and be completely engaged in your life, right up to the last breath. Who knows—perhaps, if such a place exists, you can even take it beyond into another realm. I, for one, don't want to close myself to *that* possibility— just in case it's out there waiting. The point of this whole path, indeed, is to stay open to the great mystery that you are—and keep your senses keen to the even greater mystery you may become.

Part Five

Food, Tools and Toys

Easy, Low-Fat, Old-World Recipes
for Hectic, Modern Times

FOOD IS A NATURAL EXTENSION of our female sensuality, a celebration of the fruits of the earth. It is our fuel, survival, pleasure, solace. But it can also be the ultimate entrapment, dazzling us with its delights, hitting a spot no lover can ever reach, then disappearing so fast that we're left only with its ravages, the bloating followed by emptiness. No other substance so literally becomes us or dictates how our energy will droop or soar. No other substance so clearly leaves its mark on the way we look.

Much has been made of women's obsessions with food and the cycles we ride between indulgence and denial. Many of us have slipped in and out of the black tunnels we call eating disorders. But it's not just actual anorexics, bulimics or members of Overeaters Anonymous who dance over the edge with food, eat too much, then too little, follow treats with acts of penance. As far as food is concerned, many of us have lost our balance. Creating balance is not that difficult.

We need to shift the focus away from being "victims of food" and put it back on our natural affinity for food. Women have a primal, unique history of food celebration. For centuries, we have been the dominant food gatherers and preparers. We've been the ones who cooked the meals that kept our families alive, distinguished our cultures with spicy flavors, made others feel secure in the warm vitality of our kitchens. We've learned how to ration and pace our supplies, add grains to a meat dish to make it last through a cold spell or between paychecks. We've connected our hearths to the earth, made feasts to honor the seasons— summer berries into compotes and pies, ripe tomatoes with a sprig of basil, capturing harvest in a jar. Even our bodies are like food. Children born to us ripen like large succulent fruits inside our skin and grow fat off the milk that pours from our breasts.

These days, not many of us get time in our kitchens to knead our breads and roll out our dough. Zapping dinner in the microwave after getting home from work doesn't exactly lend itself to sweet creations. Though many of us have refused to become slaves to cooking, ironically, we have become slaves somewhere else. At least the kitchen is a world we can control, if we so desire. Cooking has the power to deliver us back to a slower, natural pace, one in which flavors mature.

Personally, I've got a foot in both worlds. One half of me is the slow Buddha with a kitchen knife, humming songs while slicing onions. The other is a modern-day wild woman, careening through several universes at once. With so many worlds to conquer, who has time to cook?

The recipes in this book satisfy both ancient and modern sensibilities. All can be made in advance on a quiet Sunday and then born again, with even more flavor, throughout a week of lunches and leftovers. Or they can be whipped up quickly any time. The foods are simple, inexpensive, low-fat, delicious and substantial. There's nothing fancy, delicate or laborious here. Everything is of hardy stock: rice and beans, pasta, bread. The concept is basic—to look like a goddess, you should eat like a peasant! If it grows out of the earth, wash off the pesticides and eat it. If it comes in a box or can, read the labels carefully.

This isn't a "diet" or an extreme approach, but a way of eating that sustains long-term energy and leaves room for treats. I'm not a doctor or registered dietitian and so I leave the more detailed scientific information to those who know it best. But I cook, eat and clean. I also like to know what I'm eating and why, choosing my carbohydrates, fats and proteins wisely according to what activities I will or won't be doing, so I give myself the appropriate fuel.

Once again, the dominant principle here is to find and maintain balance—a balance of nutrients and different types of foods, as well as eating small but sufficient portions to keep energy going steady all day. The nutrients in the following recipes provide 50% to 70% carbohydrates, 15% to 35% protein, 10% to 25% fat. Although I give calories for each serving, the idea isn't to count calories, but simply be informed about which types of calories come from what sources.

There are huge areas of controversy here, such as, how much fat should we really eat? How much protein do we need? Since each of us has different requirements, there's no one answer. Proper intake depends on activity, body composition, food intolerance, and cravings. Finding the right answers for each of us takes a bit of experimentation.

However, we're all more or less in agreement about certain facts. 1) Too much fat makes us fat, contributes to elevated cholesterol, clogs arteries and increases our risk of heart disease. Yet we do need *some* fat to contribute to the formation of cell membranes and blood lipids and to synthesize vitamins. 2) Too much protein taxes the small intestine and liver and is stored as fat. Too little protein fails to provide sufficient nutrients to promote tissue growth. 3) Complex carbohydrates fuel us through life. Simple carbohydrates (such as fruit and refined sugar) take us on a quick joyride and then quickly send energy down.

Fat

The American Heart Association recommends a diet that is 30% fat. Although this represents a drop in fat consumption in the basic American diet of burgers and fries (which is 40% to 50% fat), it's still a lot of fat—and double what I like to eat. (My body functions best on approximately 60% carbs, 20% to 25% protein and 15% to 20% fat.) Doctors such as Dean Ornish in *Eat More, Weigh Less* and John MacDougal of *The MacDougal Plan*, recommend even less fat. The 30% number represents a more realistic number for people cutting back on a high-fat diet but it's not necessarily the optimal number.

If you're used to eating a lot of fat, coming off it is similar to kicking any drug. It's easier if you start by cutting the dosage gradually. You can lose the craving for the taste and sensation of fat, either by eating more complex carbohydrates or using low- or nonfat substitutes for old fattening favorites (such as nonfat cheese or nonfat frozen yogurt). Eventually, you'll get to the place where eating dense, rich fat will make you feel sick!

Fat is an energy-rich source—each gram of fat equals 9 calories. It's also a long-term investment. Only 3% of fat is used in the digestion process (compared to 20% for proteins and carbohydrates). However, it can be used wisely. A 3 P.M. snack of toast with a few slices of avocado or a smear of reduced-fat peanut butter can give you the kind of slow-burning energy necessary to get you through to dinner (much more effectively than soda and a candy bar—simple sugars which, by 3:30, will leave you even more exhausted).

Protein

Depending on what books or magazines you read, the recommended daily amounts of protein vary from 1 gram of protein per pound of body weight for "average" people to more than *4* grams per pound of body weight for hard-core bodybuilders (although that's way too much for me). It's true that weight trainers and long-distance runners (whose muscles are constantly under repair), pregnant women (the ultimate bodybuilders!) and anyone undergoing illness or rehabilitation from a physical trauma, need more of the amino acids from proteins to build and repair muscle tissue—but how much more is the great debate. Eating too much protein gives the body more than it can metabolize, so it is stored as fat. It also gives the small intestine (where protein is digested) more work than it can handle at one time. The proper amount of protein for you is an individual call—and will also change as activity changes and will increase if you put on more lean muscle mass.

Many women tend to eat too little protein, favoring carbohydrates and fat. It's a good idea to spread out moderate protein consumption throughout the day (milk with cereal, turkey in your sandwich, a nonfat yogurt snack). But within two hours *after* a weight workout it's especially important to eat protein to assist in the repair of "hungry" muscle tissue. One gram of protein equals 4 calories.

Carbohydrates

The body gets its main fuel from carbohydrates, which are sugars, whether in simple form (as in fruits and refined sugars) or complex (found in grains, potatoes, etc.). Carbohydrates offer both immediate and long-term energy. When they're absent (as in high-protein, low-carb diets), the body then switches to its backup energy source—protein. Weight loss occurs, but usually in the form of muscle, not fat. And, as any carb-depleting bodybuilder will tell you, protein isn't a very efficient energy source. (On such a diet, the brain doesn't function well—you trip over words, sidewalks, lose your keys and eventually your sanity. It's not a fun way to eat.) The moral of this story is that you need carbs to live. Carbs are also metabolized in the small intestine. When you eat more carbohydrates than you can metabolize, like protein, they're stored as fat.

If you eat 2 to 3 hours before a workout, the meal should weigh in favor of carbohydrates. If you must eat protein, keep it light and easily digestible in the form of egg whites, dairy products or liquid protein shakes. Heavy animal protein takes a while to digest and may still be in your stomach by the time you work out—not very inspirational. If you do a weight workout first thing in the morning and can't stand eating beforehand, you may "bottom out" sooner than if you forced down a small breakfast, even just a banana or a sports drink full of complex carbs. Although you're actually using up last night's dinner as your fuel source, your blood sugar may not drop as fast if you have an energy "back up" to call on once dinner is depleted. I'd recommend doing aerobics, however, on a completely empty stomach. Intense cardiovascular activity sends blood that would normally be aiding in digestion out to the heart and moving limbs. Undigested food, therefore, can sit in your stomach and make you feel sick. Also, within half an hour after a weight workout, take in about 50 grams of carbohydrates (an apple, a nonfat muffin) to replace the glycogen depleted from exercise. One gram of carbohydrates equals 4 calories.

Stocking the Kitchen

Start by getting the right foods in the house. Success is more likely when the right ingredients are on hand. Here are some essential staples to maintain a low-fat life:

grains (such as rice and barley)

pastas

nonfat cottage cheese

nonfat yogurt

nonfat milk

Weight Watchers® nonfat parmesan

balsamic and seasoned rice vinegars

salsa

low- or nonfat breads

beans (canned are okay)

water-packed white tuna

egg whites (one to four yolks per week, however, will give you extra lecithin and B vitamins)

fresh fruits (especially "slower burning" apples and bananas)

vegetables (onions, peppers, tomatoes, salad greens, carrots, broc- coli, etc.)

baking potatoes and yams

canned stewed tomatoes

corn or low-fat flour tortillas

Worcestershire sauce

tamari (soy sauce)

mustards

honey

applesauce

oatmeal

Grape Nuts® cereal

Shredded Wheat® cereal

dried fruit

popcorn (microwaved or air-popped)

rice cakes

fresh herbs and spices

Substitution

Learning to eat well is often a matter of finding substitutions for favorite foods. There are new low- and nonfat products coming out all the time. (Just beware of nonfat bakery goods that are loaded with sugar.) A little creativity in old standard recipes can cut down on fat but leave in the taste.

When a Recipe Calls For:	Use:
1 whole egg	2 egg whites
whole milk	nonfat milk or apple juice
butter for baking	water, juice, applesauce (also, carrot and apple pulp from a juicer)
oil for sautéing	broth, nonstick spray, 1 tbs. green olive oil
sour cream	nonfat sour cream, cottage cheese, or non-fat yogurt
thickeners for soup	instant or cooked potatoes, pureed squash, arrowroot, cornstarch
cheese dips	nonfat cottage cheese, whipped in food processor with spices
regular cheeses	nonfat cheeses (Some of them taste good but most don't melt as well)
tortilla chips	cut fresh tortillas, squeeze on fresh lime, bake
potato chips	potatoes sliced paper-thin, seasoned and baked

A Day in the Life

The hardest part about switching to low-fat fare is getting used to being hungry more often—and realizing that it's a good thing. It means your metabolism has sped up, which is a sign of health! You have to get over the notion that eating more makes you a "pig." You also have to plan meals a little differently—spread them out to 4 to 6 times a day, not the standard 2 or 3. It's also wise not to go hungry for too long—but carry backups at all times (rice cakes, apples, bagels, etc.) to bail out of a sugar low. Getting too hungry can be dangerous, because it will make you later inhale anything in sight.

Here's a sample menu from a day in my life. All food values were taken from standard food tables and off boxes and cans.

MEAL #1—6 A.M. Pre-workout breakfast
(2 hours before exercise, mostly carbs)

Food	Calories	Protein (grams)	Carbs (grams)	Fat (grams)
½ cup oatmeal with cinnamon, vanilla, toasted sesame seeds	155	5	27	3
¼ cup Grape Nuts	104	3	23	0
½ cup nonfat milk	48	5	7	.02*
1 banana	95	1	22.2	.2
SUBTOTAL	402	14	79.2	3.22

* even nonfat products can have trace quantities of fat.

MEAL #2—10 A.M. Post-workout meal
(protein very important)

Food	Calories	Protein (grams)	Carbs (grams)	Fat (grams)
5 scrambled egg whites	78	18	1.5	0
2 oz. salsa	21	.5	4.8	0
2 pieces whole wheat toast	128	5.8	24	1
8 oz. nonfat yogurt	128	13	18	.4
SUBTOTAL	355	37.3	48.3	1.4

MEAL #3—1 P.M. Lunch

Food	Calories	Protein (grams)	Carbs (grams)	Fat (grams)
4 oz. albacore tuna in water, with seasoned rice vinegar, nonfat cottage cheese, shredded carrot, chopped scallions, dash of Worcestershire, cracked black pepper, homemade tortilla chips and salsa				
4 oz. tuna	119	28	0	.8
1 carrot	46	1	10	.2
½ cup nonfat cottage cheese	72	14	4	0
2 corn tortillas	117	3	24	1
(heated on stove top, shredded into "chips" for scooping up tuna)				
2 oz. salsa	21	.5	4.8	0
SUBTOTAL	375	46.5	42.8	2

MEAL #4—4 P.M. Snack

Food	Calories	Protein (grams)	Carbs (grams)	Fat (grams)
1 large apple	106	.3	24	.5
2 caramel rice cakes	104	2	24	0
SUBTOTAL	210	2.3	48	.5

MEAL #5—7 P.M. Dinner

Food	Calories	Protein (grams)	Carbs (grams)	Fat (grams)
1 cup brown rice	179	4	38	1.2
⅓ cup beans	76	4.8	13.5	.3
2 oz. turkey breast, skinned, sliced, sautéed in 1 tbs. olive oil with onions in lemon, mustard and honey, dash of Worcestershire				
2 oz. turkey	105	21	0	2.3
1 tbs. olive oil	126	0	0	14
2 oz. salsa	21	.5	4.8	0
1 tbs. Weight Watchers parmesan	12	1	2	0
1 cup steamed broccoli, tossed with rice vinegar, sprinkle of toasted sesame seeds	52	4.8	7	.5
Dessert	50	.3	11.5	.3
½ cup hot applesauce, with cinnamon				
⅛ cup raisins	71	.8	17	0
SUBTOTAL	692	37.2	93.8	18.6
DAILY TOTAL	2034	137.3	312.1	25.72

To find out the percentages of carbs, proteins and fats in total calories, use some simple math. Since one gram of protein and one gram of carbohydrates each equals 4 calories, multiply those total grams by 4:

$137.3 \times 4 = 549.2$ total calories from protein

$312.1 \times 4 = 1248.4$ total calories from carbohydrates

And since one gram of fat equals 9 calories, multiply the total fat grams times 9.

$25.72 \times 9 = 231.48$ calories from fat

These numbers should add up to your total calories; but don't worry if you're off by a few percentage points or whole numbers. The numbers listed in food tables or on boxes and cans aren't always totally accurate.

Also, to simplify the math, you may want to round up or down to the nearest whole.

Next, divide each of those last total numbers by the daily total calories.

549.2 divided by 2034 = .27 or 27% calories from protein

1248.4 divided by 2034 = .613 or 61% calories from carbohydrates

231.48 divided by 2034 = .114 or almost 12% of calories from fat

(This is a very low-fat day. To add fat, spread 1 tbs. reduced-fat peanut butter on nonfat bread, for 7.5 grams of fat (7.5 × 9 = 67.50 more calories from fat). This will also add 4.5 grams of protein and 6 grams of carbohydrates.

Recipes

GALLO PINTO OR FANCY RICE AND BEANS

(Translated from Spanish, this means "spotted rooster," since it's spotted like a rooster's tail.)

This recipe comes from my mother-in-law, Yelba Nunez, from Nicaragua, who cooks much the same way as did Tita in the novel *Like Water for Chocolate*. The secret of this and all recipes, says Yelba, is to cook "con amor" (with love)—for that is the only way to release the magical flavors from the humblest meal.

One good vat of beans and rice can last for days and live many lives in tacos, burritos, omelets and salads. This version is tasty and highly nutritious.

INGREDIENTS:

2 cups dry black beans (or two cans cooked black beans)

3 cups white or brown rice (or mix together)

1 green pepper

2 red onions

Salsa (jarred is fine)

TO COOK:

Rinse, sort and soak beans for an hour or two—not overnight. After too much time, they begin to ferment, and that's what causes intestinal gas. Rinse and cover with fresh water, then cook at a slow boil about 1¼ hours. Chop a green pepper, add to uncooked rice, add water and cook (a rice cooker makes it perfect every time). In a regular saucepan, after you put the rice in the pan, cover it with 6 cups of water (for grains, it's always 1 part grain, 2 parts water), start in cold water on medium heat and try to resist opening the lid for 30 minutes. Then check, fluff, and stir.

In a large frying pan, sauté the red onion in 1 tbs. olive oil (the fragrant green kind). Add beans and rice. Once both are cooked (and here's where the love comes in), *gently* fold together, careful not to cut up the rice. Add a bit of the liquid from the beans to color the rice a light brown.

TO SERVE:

Top with Worcestershire sauce, salsa, 1 tbs. Weight Watchers parmesan and, if available, any leftover chicken breast or turkey.

Heat 2 corn tortillas with no oil in a hot iron skillet or directly on a gas burner (watch that it doesn't catch on fire). Brown, flip and serve. Scoop up gallo pinto with bits of tortilla. Deliciosa!

1 serving

	Calories	Protein	Carbs	Fat
1 onion	67	2.5	13.7	.2
1 tbs. olive oil	126	0	0	14
1 cup white rice	158	3	36	.2
⅓ cup beans	76	4.8	13.5	.3
2 oz. salsa	21	.5	4.8	0
1 tbs. Weight Watchers parmesan	12	1	2	0
2 corn tortillas	117	3	24	1
TOTAL	577	14.8	94	15.7

$14.8 \times 4 = 59.2$ calories from protein

59.2 divided by 577 (total calories) = .10 or 10% calories from protein

$94 \times 4 = 376$ calories from carbohydrates

376 divided by 577 = .65 or 65% calories from carbohydrates

$15.7 \times 9 = 141.3$ calories from fats

141.3 divided by 577 = .245 or 25% calories from fat

(If you want to make this a nearly nonfat treat, sauté the onion with no oil, just two plum tomatoes.)

TURKEY BURGERS

Sometimes there's nothing like a burger. These are not only lean and light, but have only half the animal protein of a regular burger.

INGREDIENTS:

*Approx. 1 lb. 100% skinned turkey
  breast, ground
1 cup leftover rice
chopped bell pepper
seasonings to taste:
1 tbs. tamari*

*1 tbs. Worcestershire sauce
For a nuttier burger, add:
  2 tbs. roasted sunflower seeds
  1 cup kidney or garbanzo beans,
  coarsely ground*

TO PREPARE:

Mash up beans and rice in food processor, adding a bit of salsa to liquefy. In a big mixing bowl, combine rice and bean mixture with chopped turkey until well mixed. Form into patties (makes approx. 6 large patties). Coat pan with nonstick spray and cook on medium heat (these are a bit too crumbly to make on a barbecue). Cover and flip to cook both sides.

Serve on a bagel or bun and garnish with mustard, salsa, tomato, lettuce, and/or nonfat Thousand Island dressing.

1 serving (1 pattie)

	Calories	Protein	Carbs	Fat
2 oz. turkey	105	21	0	2.3
⅙ cup white rice	25	.25	6	
⅙ cup beans	39	2.4	6.8	.2
1 burger bun	118	3.3	21.2	2.2
TOTALS	287	26.95	34	4.7

26.95 × 4 = 107.8 calories from protein

107.8 divided by 287 = .375 or 38% calories from protein

34 × 4 = 136 calories from carbohydrates

136 divided by 287 = .47 or 47% calories from carbohydrates

4.7 × 9 = 42.3 calories from fat

42.3 divided by 287 = .147 or 15% calories from fat

KAREN'S INCREDIBLE CAESAR SALAD

This salad is as sweet as candy. I could eat huge bowls of it!

INGREDIENTS:

1 head romaine lettuce
4 pieces nonfat bread, toasted
1 red onion

a sprinkle of toasted sesame seeds
4 tbs. Weight Watchers parmesan
1 can kidney beans

Wash and dry lettuce. Chop into edible sizes. Sauté onion in nonstick pan until brown and "marbled." Toast nonfat bread and cut into crouton-sized cubes. Add all ingredients to salad bowl.

THE DRESSING:

½ cup seasoned rice vinegar
½ cup nonfat cottage cheese

1 tsp. mustard
1 tsp honey
¼ bunch of scallions

Whip together in a food processor and store in a jar in the refrigerator (you've got plenty for two big salads). Toss salad, sprinkling with sesame seeds and nonfat parmesan. Serves 4.

Per serving

	Calories	Protein	Carbs	Fat
Salad:				
2 cups romaine lettuce	23	1.4	4	.2
¼ onion	17	.6	3.4	.2
1 slice nonfat bread	48	2	10	0
¼ cup kidney beans	62	3.5	12	0
Dressing per serving:				
approx. 4 tbs. seasoned rice vinegar	48	0	12	0
⅛ cup nonfat cottage cheese	17	3.3	1	0
1 tbs. Weight Watchers parmesan	12	1	2	0
trace mustard and sesame, scallions and honey	14			1.5
TOTAL	241	11.8	44.4	1.9

11.8 × 4 = 47.2 calories from protein

47.2 divided by 241 = .19 or 19% calories from protein

44.4 × 4 = 177.6 calories from carbohydrates

177.6 divided by 241 = .736 or 74% calories from carbs

1.9 × 9 = 17.1 calories from fat

17.1 divided by 241 = .07 or 7% calories from fat

EGG WHITE FRITATA

Egg white omelets can be very fluffy and delicious with the right spices. To give eggs more color, density and lecithin, add one yolk per 4 to 6 whites.

INGREDIENTS:

1 onion, chopped and sautéed
½ cup stewed tomatoes
or 3 plum tomatoes chopped and
*   sautéed*
8 egg whites
nonfat jack, cheddar or parmesan
*   cheese*

A choice of spices:
*   chili powder*
*   fresh thyme*
*   fresh oregano*
*   chopped scallions*
*   chopped cilantro*

TO PREPARE:

In a nonstick pan, or omelet pan coated with nonstick spray, sauté onions and peppers until slightly browned. Add tomatoes and cook some more. Separate egg yolks from whites and whip whites until foamy. Pour into pan, add cheese and spices. Scramble a bit to make omelet thicker. Cover and cook. Flip to cook some more. Cut in half. Sprinkle with salsa, Tabasco, more nonfat cheese, fresh scallions, etc. Serves 2. Serve with toast or corn tortillas.

1 serving

	Calories	Protein	Carbs	Fat
4 egg whites	61	14	1.2	0
½ onion	36	1.2	6.8	.4
1 oz. nonfat cheese	40	8	1	.4
3 plum tomatoes	28	2.4	3.3	.6
1 tbs. Weight Watchers parmesan	12	1	2	0
2 pieces whole wheat toast	128	5.8	24	1
TOTALS	305	32.4	38.3	2.4

$32.4 \times 4 = 129.6$ calories from protein

129.6 divided by $305 = .424$ or 4% calories from protein

$38.3 \times 4 = 153.2$ calories from carbohydrates

153.2 divided by $305 = .50$ or 50% calories from carbs

$2.4 \times 9 = 21.6$ calories from fat

21.6 divided by $305 = .07$ or 7% calories from fat

PASTA CON FRIJOLES

No one ever seems to get sick of pasta. This is a great stand-by, simple dinner.

INGREDIENTS FOR MARINARA SAUCE:

1 onion
1 pepper
1 28-oz. can stewed tomatoes
1 cup applesauce
4 to 6 extra plum tomatoes to make
  chunkier, if desired
1 can kidney or white beans
A choice of spices:
  fresh basil
  fresh oregano
  a dash of balsamic vinegar,
    mustard, garlic

Options to add protein to sauce:
  100% ground turkey breast (2 oz.
    per serving)
  skinned, boneless chicken breast, 1
    per person
  1 cup nonfat cottage cheese,
    whipped in food processor and
    added to sauce for a tomato-
    based cream sauce
or 6 scrambled egg whites, cooked
    separately and added into
    sauce

TO PREPARE:

Sauté onion, pepper, tomatoes. Add turkey or chicken to cooked onions and peppers and brown. Add stewed tomatoes and applesauce and let turkey or chicken cook in the sauce. (Or spoon in whipped cottage cheese or precooked scrambled eggs for additional protein.) Add cooked beans and spices. Serves 6 to 8.

Cook pasta (no oil necessary in water if pasta is stirred frequently). Drain. Toss with 4 tbs. sweetened rice vinegar to keep pasta from sticking together, especially good for leftovers. Pour sauce on top.

Per serving

	Calories	*Protein*	*Carbs*	*Fat*
2 cups cooked spaghetti	321	6	72	1
4 tbs. rice vinegar	48	0	12	0
Sauce: (with turkey breast)				
½ cup stewed tomatoes	40	1	9	0
¼ cup applesauce	24	0	6	0
¼ onion	17	.6	3.4	.2
¼ cup kidney beans	62	3.5	12	0
2 oz. 100% ground turkey				
breast	105	21	0	2.3
TOTALS	617	32.1	114.4	3.5

$32.1 \times 4 = 128.4$ calories from protein

128.4 divided by $617 = .208$ or 21% calories from protein

$114.4 \times 4 = 457.6$ calories from carbs

457.6 divided by $617 = .74$ or 74% of calories from carbs

$3.5 \times 9 = 31.5$ calories from fat

31.5 divided by $617 = .05$ or 5% calories from fat

Foods to Eat When You're on the Go

turkey sandwich with mustard, lettuce and tomato—hold the mayo

tuna pita—also hold the mayo

leftover pasta—toss with rice vinegar, chicken chunks, spices

bagels

bananas, oranges or apples

quick snacks:

caramel flavored rice cakes

nonfat yogurt—frozen or regular

breadsticks

air-popped popcorn

Maintenance Tips

- Eat small meals or snacks throughout the day to keep energy fairly constant. I like the "fist method" of distinguishing a snack from a meal. A snack is the size of one fist, a meal two.

- Cook food yourself as much as possible and take it with you. Invest in plastic containers and a cooler.

- When eating in restaurants, order suspicious sauces on the side. Order grilled rather than sautéed entrees. Never eat anything fried. Tell them to hold the cream, sour cream and cheese.

- On airplanes, call ahead and order the low-fat entree. Some are actually good.

- Make room for occasional treats—a piece of chocolate, a shared dessert, 93% fat-free hot fudge on nonfat frozen yogurt.

- Eat a polite-sized portion of a fat-laden meal at a friend's house. It won't kill you. Start the next day with a bowl of oatmeal to get it moving on out!

- Beware of the special relationship. When you have to have it every day and use it as a reward, you've entered the land of addiction. Be a good addict and give or throw it away. If it's not in the cabinet, it won't call your name.

It's a Jungle Out There

Although things are looking up for the health-conscious who yearn to travel unencumbered through the world, it's still tough to maintain a low-fat way of life. It's not safe to eat what many so innocently offer. Even the low-fat, natural and "lite" products are highly suspect. (Read the labels and do the math. Multiply the fat grams by 9 and compare against the total calories to determine if it's truly low in fat.) The predators—fat, oversized portions, sugar and alcohol—are coiled behind every rock, waiting to yank you off course. Even mothers and grandmothers practice temptation, pushing greasy roasts, buttery potatoes, kugels, pastries—taking all your protests about fat as personal insults to their cooking.

Keeping a commitment to yourself without upsetting other people is quite a challenge. It threatens them by making them "wrong" for having their eating habits while holding you up as a superior human being—even though that isn't your intention at all. Many people do not understand that eating this way is a choice, not a hardship. They also fail to realize that:

1. You probably eat more total calories than they do. So, no you don't eat like a bird.

2. When you eat a fat-rich meal, it tends to stick in the gut like poison. (This doesn't happen to people who eat this way all the time—at least, they don't notice it as much.)

3. You're the one who has to work it off.

Making a lifestyle choice often leaves others behind. As your body improves and your enthusiasm soars, be conscious of others' feelings.

It's wise to practice discretion regarding your eating habits and be silent with your judgment of others'—even when they're vocal about yours. That may be hard especially if someone you love eats too much fat or diets to extremes. In such a case, try speaking your opinion quickly, firmly, just once without begging. People are more inclined to follow your example if you don't cram your opinions down their throats.

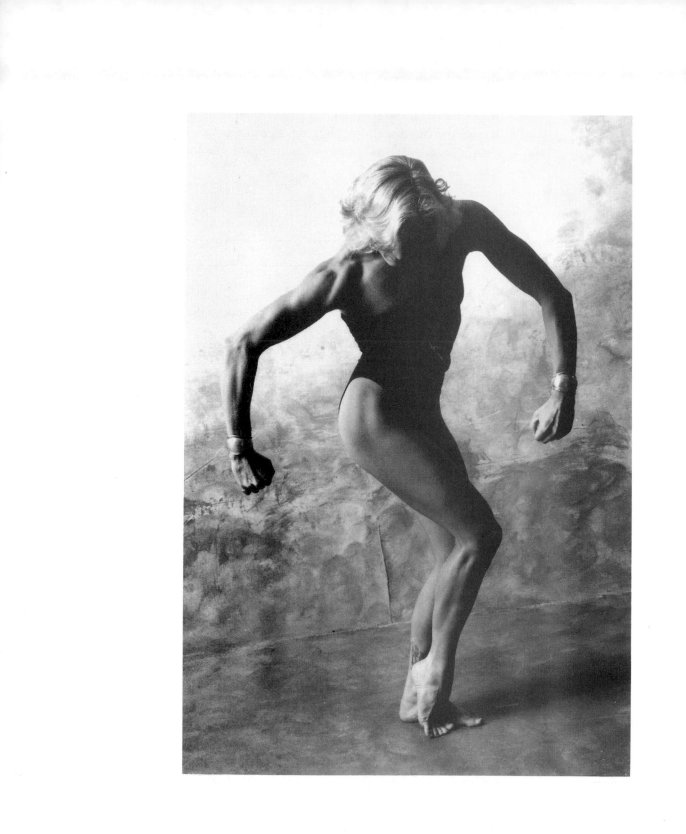

Meditation for the
Fully Realized Woman

I AM A BEAUTIFUL WOMAN, with a beauty that doesn't wash off. I earned it, unearthed it, rescued it like a jewel in the dust, picked it up and made it shine.

For years, I did not see it, though I sensed it was there. Now it dazzles and thrives.

I am healthy, capable, independent, strong yet still so fragile, floored by a sigh. My body is that of a creator—angles meeting curves, hardness drifting into soft.

I am mother, daughter, sister, lover to myself. Embraccable and brave, I extend my heart.

My body is my home, my home a shrine to life, comfortable, warm and rich with treasures. Mine is the scent of hot spices caught in a breeze, mine the laughter that wings through the door. I share myself only with those who honor me as I am and protect myself, my house and my time from invaders.

I search for my center in the midst of chaos, practice peace as wild dogs clamor in my mind. I use power for the greater good, release rage in neutral settings, with no one innocent in the line of fire.

I am learning how to persist and when to let go, am willing to feel all emotions to their depths and exaltations, to wake up in every nerve and no longer am afraid of my life.

Both my beauty and strength transcend age, time and perhaps even this lifetime.

Each day I am new, yet more at home in myself. Moment by moment, I create my world.

More Tools and Toys
for Transformation

I F YOU CAN'T or don't want to join a gym, get yourself a set of dumbbells—2, 5, 8, 10, 15, 20, 25 lbs. and possibly higher, plus a pair of ankle weights, 1 to 5 lbs. each (the average is 2½, many come with adjustable weights). That, plus standing leg work with or without weights, will see you through many of the exercises in this book.

Dyna-bands also work as inexpensive, convenient, portable alternatives to weights—and in many cases offer a greater challenge than light weights since they give more resistance through a greater r.o.m. Many of the free-weight and cable exercises here can be adapted to bands. Dyna-bands come in 3- or 4-foot pre-cut lengths or in bulk rolls you cut yourself. They also come in four strengths:

- pink—easy

- green or blue—moderate

- purple or yellow—challenging

- gray—tough!

Available from Fitness Wholesale, 1-800-537-5512
My video *Dyna-Gym* shows a full band workout—good for beginners

and intermediates—and shows the connection between bands and weights. This 43-minute workout includes window inserts that show:

- How to do the same exercises with weights

- Common mistakes to avoid

$24.95 suggested retail. Comes with two 4-foot green Dyna-bands—an $8.00 value. Available through:

- ExerScience Stores and Catalogues, a division of Nordic Track

- Collage Video Catalogue, 1-800-433-6769

- Fitness Wholesale, 1-800-537-5512

Also by Karen

Cher's Body Confidence video—Second half of tape features a 40-minute band workout, one-on-one in black mesh, with Cher.

DEEP-WATER AQUATIC EXERCISE

- *The Aquajogger Deep Water Workout* with Karen Andes

- *Aquajive* audio cassette with Karen Andes

Aquajogger flotation belts available through Excel Sports Science, 1-800-922-9544
Instructor discounts available through Fitness Wholesale

MORE AQUATIC EQUIPMENT

- A full line of aquatic exercise equipment including webbed gloves, buoyant ankle cuffs, dumbbells and more, available through Fitness Wholesale, 1-800-537-5512

- The "Aquatunes Belt," a waterproof, submersible pouch for a portable cassette player. Earphones are submersible, too, so you can listen to music while you swim. (Put cassette player in a "Ziploc" bag for double protection.) $39.95 at Excel Sports Science, 1-800-922-9544.

Videos

Collage Video Catalogue (1-800-433-6769) stocks one of the most complete selections of exercise videos. Collage carefully screens each tape, gives full descriptions and makes suggestions (and in some cases, tells you what to avoid). Some of the harder-to-find tapes are here, made by top-notch instructors who lack large distributors. An excellent resource for all sorts of workouts.

Inversion Equipment

Gravity Plus catalogue shows a full array of equipment to let you "take a load" off your back—and hang at your comfort level. Very creative, longevity-enhancing aids include:

- Back swings
- Physioballs (giant rubber balls for spine stabilization and stretching)
- Inversion Swings
- Body Bridge
- The Back Bubble
- "Nada" Chair Back support system (a portable lower back support "strap" that goes around back and knees; great for sitting at desks, long car or plane rides).

Gravity Plus Catalogue, 1-800-383-8056

References

B ECAUSE MY QUEST for strength and motion has been so long and ongoing, it's tough to crystallize into a bibliography all the sources that contributed to this work. This isn't just the result of studying physical movement—but also how words dance on a page, how knowledge penetrates the mind, how we truly learn, synthesize and then create a form of our own.

Although some of these books are not directly related to physical strength, all of them have had an impact on my thoughts.

The Body

Juhan, Deane. *Job's Body.* New York: Station Hill Press, 1987.

Leonard, George. *The Ultimate Athlete.* New York: Viking, 1975.

Smith, Edward W. L., Ph.D. *Not Just Pumping Iron, On the Psychology of Lifting Weights.* Springfield, IL: Charles C. Thomas, 1989.

Hatfield, Fred. *Bodybuilding, A Scientific Approach.* Chicago: Contemporary Books, 1984.

Jordan, Peg. *Fitness Theory & Practice.* Sherman Oaks, CA: AFAA and Reebok University, 1993.

Tesch, Per, and Gary Dudley. *Muscle Meets Magnet.* Stockholm, Sweden: PA Tesch, AB, 1993.

Kapit, Wynn, and Lawrence Elson. *The Anatomy Coloring Book.* New York: Harper & Row, 1977.

Murphy, Michael. *The Future of the Body*. Los Angeles: Jeremy P. Tarcher, Inc., 1992.

Dobson, Terry, and Victor Miller. *Aikido in Everyday Life*. Berkeley, CA: North Atlantic Books, 1978.

The Mind

Leonard, George. *Mastery*. New York: Penguin, 1991.

Heider, John. *The Tao of Leadership*. New York: Bantam, 1986.

Roth, Gabrielle. *Maps To Ecstasy*. San Rafael, CA: New World Library, 1989.

The Evolution of Spirit

Pierrakos, Eva. *The Pathwork of Self Transformation*. New York: Bantam, 1980.

Williamson, Marianne. *A Return to Love*. New York: HarperCollins, 1992.

Brennan, Barbara. *Hands of Light*. New York: Bantam, 1988.

Women

Williamson, Marianne. *A Woman's Worth*. New York: Random House, 1993.

Pinkola-Estes, Clarissa. *Women Who Run With the Wolves*. New York: Ballantine Books, 1992.

Woolf, Virginia. *A Room of One's Own*. New York: Harcourt Brace Jovanovich, 1981.

Shinoda-Bolen, Jean. *Goddesses in Every Woman*. New York: Harper & Row, 1985.

Wolf, Naomi. *The Beauty Myth*. New York: Doubleday, 1991.

Food

Ornish, Dean. *Eat More, Weigh Less*. New York: HarperCollins, 1993.

MacDougal, John, and Mary MacDougal. *The MacDougal Plan*. New Jersey: New Win Publishing Inc., 1983.